# Counseling and Spirituality

## Views from the Profession

Oliver Morgan

Editor

**LAHASKA PRESS**

Houghton Mifflin Company    Boston   New York

*To my professional mentors in the arts of healing and clinical theology:*
*Merle Jordan, Chris Schlauch, Homer Jernigan, Gene Abroms, and*
*Ivan Boszormenyi-Nagy.*
*and*
*To my wife, Ellen:*
*My anchor and soul-mate,*
*my mentor and partner*
*in a new life of intimacy and care,*
*and rich spiritual blessings.*

Publisher, Lahaska Press: Barry Fetterolf
Senior Editor, Lahaska Press: Mary Falcon
Editorial Assistant: Evangeline Bermas
Senior Project Editor: Kimberly Gavrilles
Art and Design Manager: Gary Crespo
Composition Buyer: Chuck Dutton
Associate Manufacturing Buyer: Brian Pieragostini
Director of Sales and Marketing, Lahaska Press: Heather Murray

Cover image © stamm2004/theispot.com

For instructors who want more information about Lahaska Press books and teaching aids, contact the Houghton Mifflin Faculty Services Center at
Tel: 800-733-1717, x4034
Fax: 800-733-1810
Or visit us on the Web at **www.lahaskapress.com**.

Printed in the U.S.A.

Library of Congress Control Number: 2006925457

ISBN-10: 0-618-47494-3
ISBN-13: 978-0-618-47494-3

123456789-EB-10 09 08 07 06

# Contents

CHAPTER FOUR

## Seven Stages of Spiritual Development: A Framework to Solve Psycho-Spiritual Problems    64

### Daya Singh Sandhu

CHAPTER FIVE

## Weaving Sacred Threads into Multicultural Counseling    93

### Mary A. Fukuyama

CHAPTER SIX

## Breath of Heaven    110

### Craig S. Cashwell

APPENDIX A

## ASERVIC Competencies for Integrating Spirituality into Counseling

❧

# Preface

"We are spiritual beings with specifically local experiences."
—R. Wubbolding (2000), *Reality Therapy for the 21st Century*

This book is intended to fill a gap in the growing literature on spirituality and counseling.

Interest in spirituality has been intensifying in the United States for some time now. Newspapers, magazines, websites, talk shows, published surveys, government reports, and a host of other venues have contributed to the conversation. A number of publications, both popular and scholarly, have addressed the topic in relation to health generally as well as physical wellness, aging and care for the elderly, alcohol and other drug abuse, disabilities, and a host of societal issues from corporate management and organizational life to coping with cancer, from changing careers to living in families, from working with the poor and marginalized to ecological concerns and care for the earth.

Across the range of health-related fields there has been a growing body of scholarship that connects interest in spirituality and developing a spiritual life with a variety of clinical concerns and approaches. Social work (Abels, 2000; Canda, 1998; Canda & Smith, 2001) and nursing (Barnum, 2003; Taylor, 2001) have added important scholarship in this area. Physician trainers in medical schools and residency programs, along with those who develop medical school curricula, have focused attention on the topic (Koenig, 2002; Jonas & Levin, 1999; Levin, 2002; Larson, Lu, & Swyers, 1997; Shea, 2000; Shelly, 2000).

In addition, some well-known names in contemporary clinical psychology and psychotherapy have conducted research into spiritual issues and published important studies on integrating spirituality and clinical practice (Miller, 1999; Pargament, 1997; Richards & Bergin, 1997; Shafranske, 1996). Several important journals in psychology, including the *American Psychologist* (Volume 58 (1), January 2003) as well as the *Monitor on Psychology* (Volume 34 (11), December 2003), have published

articles and special issues in this field. The literature of family therapy
has seen a similar increase in scholarly and clinical attention with books
and journal articles (Frame, 2000; Jordan, 1999; Walsh, 1999) as well
as special issues of the *Journal of Marital and Family Therapy* (Volume 26
(2), April 2000) and professional magazines such as the *Family Therapy
Magazine* (September–October, 2003).

There is a similar story of emerging and sustained interest in spirituality among professional counselors and psychotherapists. A number
of book-length publications have appeared, and there appears to be no
shortage of additional books in the wings (Burke & Miranti, 1995;
Frame, 2003; Fukuyama & Sevig, 1999; Kelly, 1995). Professional as-
sociations, such as the Association for Spiritual, Ethical, and Religious
Values in Counseling (ASERVIC), publish "White Papers" and lists of
"competencies" for spiritually-focused counseling and clinical work (see,
for example, *http://www.aservic.org/new_page_1.htm*). A number of special-
ized practice areas within the profession of counseling also have a history
of attention to the topic. These include addictions counseling (Clinebell,
1998; Morgan & Jordan, 1999; Ringwald, 2002) and rehabilitation
counseling (Gaventa & Coulter, 2002; VandeCreek, 1999; Vash, 1994).
A 1995 special double issue of the journal *Rehabilitation Education* appeared with a variety of articles discussing the integration of spirituality
within the theories and practices of that discipline (Vash & McCarthy,
1995). The journal *Professional School Counseling* also has a special issue on
the topic (Volume 7(5), June 2004).

In short, contemporary awareness, conversation, and publication
around the issue of spirituality and its integration with clinical practice
are sustained and increasing. It is no wonder that the advent of spiritual
concerns within counseling has been hailed as a new "5th Force" movement (Stanard, Sandhu, & Painter, 2000), complementing previous
"movements" such as humanistic and multicultural concerns.

I have been attentive to these developments for some time. As a professional counselor educator, marital and family therapist, pastoral psychotherapist, and ordained person, I have watched the growing interest
in spirituality and the clinical disciplines—as we shall soon see, part of
a wider movement within American culture—with delight, and I have
tried to make my own small contributions to this growth over the years
(Morgan, 1987, 1989, 2000, 2002a & b).

As I read the current situation, professional counselors, counselor educators, and practicing psychotherapists are now ready to move more
directly from theory-to-practice in this new field. The literature has
reached a point of maturity where justifying the integration of spirituality

within counseling and psychotherapy is no longer needed and where various distinctions and cautions are well understood. Many of our colleagues "get it" and are willing to believe that the integration can be part of "best practices" and is valuable to clients. What are needed now are models of application, both for students and for seasoned practitioners, and encouragement to begin the task.

Discussions of competencies for integrating counseling and spirituality refer, as they do in the multicultural arena, to the practitioner acquiring "self-awareness, knowledge and skills" as essential elements in competent practice (Sue, Arredondo, & McDavis, 1992). How do we make these competencies come alive for someone who wants to try? How do we present models for this kind of professional development and practice? Here is the current need that this book attempts to address.

In May of 2003, I contacted a number of professional counselors who had published in the area of spirituality and counseling and whose writings indicated that they were continuing to integrate spiritual concerns and values into their professional practice. Many of them I had met or worked with previously, and I had attended workshops and presentations they had given in earlier years. They represented a variety of specialties within professional counseling such as community or school counseling, rehabilitation or multicultural counseling, and work with addictions.

My proposal was simple: Would they be willing to write and publish a book chapter that captured their *experience* of integrating spiritual concerns into their clinical and professional work? It seemed to me that a sufficient base of knowledge had been laid. What were needed were models of how this integration might occur and a sharing of experience that might encourage others who were willing to attempt the task. I wanted them to address the question: How *does* someone accomplish this integration in practice? What does it look like?

As I discussed the project with colleagues and sent letters of invitation to potential contributors, however, I became increasingly aware of the "adventure" I was inviting them to join. First of all, I wanted them to hew close to their own experience in presenting their points of view. I believed (and still do!) that the story of their own interest in the subject and their real-life attempts to bring these spiritual interests into their counseling rooms was a tale worth telling. Second, I wanted them to give us a glimpse of their actual work with clients so that readers could see how this kind of integration can be accomplished.

Students, and even experienced clinicians, often benefit from such a glimpse into the counseling room. Consequently, I asked each contributor to provide a chapter that included (a) his or her view of spirituality and how it relates to counseling practice, (b) a narrative of his or her own personal and professional journey to seeing the importance of this issue, and (c) a case description, including a brief verbatim or transcript, that demonstrated how spiritual issues or concerns could be included in counseling encounters. My hope was that such a publication would help counseling students and professionals alike.

Every person (!) I contacted was willing to work on the project and communicated back to me how the approach I was suggesting stimulated them. Each person's enthusiasm confirmed my belief in the project's overall design and my desire to complete the project. However, the contributors were also a bit anxious and, over the course of the writing and revision process, contacted me numerous times to let me know just how demanding the task was.

Many of the contributors are not only practicing clinicians but are also counselor educators. They are practiced at communicating in specific ways; they are social scientist–practitioners who teach and write in conformity to certain "rules of the road." They are, in short, professors. Professors! And, there's the rub.

Academic writing tends to rely on analysis and distinctions; it often values experience-distant judgments and presentations of theory-laden material that is amply cited and referenced. It collates the knowledge gleaned from others and attempts to keep one's own biases at bay while searching for the truth of a matter. While the clinical academic writer's own experience is underneath the writing, there are conventions for presenting case material and drawing conclusions that can then be confirmed by well-cited comparisons to the work of others. Academic writing is, in short, rarely personal and experiential, rarely subjective.

However, I was asking my contributors to write in just that way, which was something quite different from their usual "comfort zone." I *wanted* a more intimate and engaging book. I was asking them to write about their own ideas, their own personal journey of discovery, and their sense of why this topic was important. I was asking not so much for a review of the literature, but for a recounting of their own individual narrative of discovery—a presentation of their own thinking and practice, personal choices, professional preferences, and concrete experience. I wanted them to share *themselves* with us. I was asking them to write about their own cases and reveal for wider consumption the way they work in the consulting room. I wanted them to be professionally transparent, which would in turn allow us to enter into the intimacy of encounters with clients. I was requesting that they be much more self-revealing than is often the case in traditional scholarship.

The task was challenging, but I believe each one of the contributors gave it his or her best. I am indebted to each one for the willingness to commit time and energy to the project. They endured frequent communications and suggestions from me and several rounds of revision. Their egos did not get in the way of accepting and hearing some pretty straightforward editorial advice. I hope they feel their final product was better and richer because of the process. They have made a significant contribution to our understanding of spirituality and, in particular, to the incorporation of spiritual themes, ideas, and activities into the best practices of our profession. Their willingness to explore their own journey of self-awareness, knowledge acquisition, and skill development, along with their openness about actual practice, give us models of courageous and generous collaboration.

## The Organization of This Book

In the initial chapters, I try to set a context for the rest of the book and the contributors' chapters that follow. I wanted to lay out a brief history of the topic and remind readers that the integration of counseling and spirituality has followed a winding, and sometimes contentious, path. These two fields of endeavor have not always been interested in each other (to say the least!), and today's willingness to work together is still something of a new venture. I also wanted to offer the reader a model or template for the rest of the book. As I've said, I knew I was asking the contributors to do something new and challenging, and I thought it was only fair to try my hand at it first.

Chapter 1 is intentionally different from the other chapters. It briefly depicts the history of counseling and spirituality as I see it and suggests several contemporary influences that help to explain why these two disciplines are interested in—and indeed, need—each other. I have been able to identify ten such influences; the reader may come up with more. This chapter also contains my attempt to discuss the notion of spirituality used in the book. Then, in Chapter 2, I present my own way of conducting and thinking about the integration of spirituality with counseling. In as clear a way as possible, I try to discuss issues of counselor identity and the "spiritual platform" of my practice, while providing a more concrete sense of spirituality as I understand it and try to live it, personally and professionally. The case of Richard provides some measure of concreteness as I try to demonstrate moving from theory-to-practice. I hope this chapter gives the reader a more concrete sense of what is to follow from others.

The remaining chapters contain offerings from ten professional counselors, women and men whose specialties cover a variety of counseling
approaches as well as a diverse set of spiritual paths and religious traditions. Community, school, rehabilitation, addictions, collegiate, and
multicultural counseling are all represented. A diverse set of Eastern
spiritual approaches as well as Native American and traditional Christian
approaches are presented as well.

In Chapter 3 "Ford" Brooks provides us with insights from the world
of addiction counseling and elaborates his perspective in the case study
of Spencer, a recovering alcoholic. Ford's own family story and spiritual
journey are compelling and, while his religious roots are pretty traditional, there is an individuality to Ford's journey that is all his own. For
those interested in a "spirituality of the outdoors," his chapter provides
some interesting affirmation.

I was delighted when Daya Singh Sandhu agreed to contribute a chapter, and his offering (Chapter 4) does not disappoint. His experience as
a practitioner of the Sikh spiritual tradition allows him to look at the integration of counseling and spirituality from a unique vantage point. His
integration of this view within a seven-stage developmental perspective,
and his generous willingness to share his *Experience Based Spiritual Development Scale (EBSDS)* with our readers, is a two-fold bonus. The reader
also benefits from seeing these spiritual elements applied to the case of
Carolyn, and suggestions are made for how to incorporate developmental
aspects of her autobiography into spiritually-sensitive counseling.

Mary Fukuyama's (Chapter 5) family experience as a "preacher's kid"
and her multicultural experience of mixed ethnicity (Japanese and Anglo-
American), colored with experiences of racism, provide a rich and fertile
ground for her view of spirituality and its possibilities in counseling practice. Identifying herself as a "global citizen" and an explorer of various
spiritual paths, she presents a case of a female graduate student exploring
and questioning her spiritual beliefs (Buddhist/Zen) in the face of grief
and loss. Her section of Recommendations for those who wish to integrate counseling and spirituality is well worth reading and pondering.

In Chapter 6, titled "Breath of Heaven," Craig Cashwell gives us several ways to be helpful in the counseling room by presenting his own
use of multiple spiritual strategies. In particular, his incorporation of
contemplative prayer and therapeutic breathwork into the case of Sara,
an educated woman searching for a deeper spiritual life, challenges us
to imagine new possibilities in the integration of counseling and spirituality. His Recommendations for those who might wish to try their
hand at this integration are simple and straightforward. His review of

breathwork principles can serve as a practical introduction to this spiritual practice and its potential integration into counseling.

Chapter 7 by Rebecca Powell Stanard is perhaps the most poetic of the chapters. She beautifully lays out a worldview that is rooted in Buddhist practice and an accepting clinical approach grounded in person-centered commitments. In the case she presents, her integration of these elements reflects a kind of powerful and yet tranquil beauty. The commonplace tools that are utilized—good theory, journaling, ritual, creative arts—are reframed as familiar yet deeply spiritual interventions.

To some extent, every spirituality lives at the intersection of worldview, lifestyle, and specific practices. In Chapter 8, Michael Tlanusta Garrett, a counselor educator and member of the Eastern Band of the Cherokee Nation, provides a tantalizing glimpse into the worldview of Native American traditions. His story and the chapter that emerges from it raise fascinating questions about the integration of counseling approaches in a more earth-friendly, spiritual way.

Richard Watts—counselor educator, ordained pastor, Adlerian psychotherapist, and self-described "traditional Christian"—presents a challenging case example of when clients' spiritual or religious perspective *is* part of the problem. Readers will, I believe, be fascinated by the paradoxical yet sensitive way in which Richard works with the couple he presents in Chapter 9.

Mary Alice Bruce, a good friend and leader in counselor education from the University of Wyoming, generously responded when I asked her, late in the project, to contribute. In Chapter 10, she provides us with a model of gentle grace and depth as she explores the role of spirituality in work as a school counselor educator. While some of the issues facing school counselors might seem to limit their integration of spirituality, Mary Alice shows a genial way to incorporate spiritual development through group work that nurtures students' awareness, self-knowledge, and acceptance of self and others.

Disability, like addiction or a peak experience, can often be a privileged (yet disguised) pathway to deeper spiritual integration. I knew this book needed a contribution from rehabilitation counseling, and Henry McCarthy has provided that gift in Chapter 11. He has found a kind of resonance within his practice of Unitarian Universalism, his commitments as a conscientious objector and social justice advocate, and his profession of rehabilitation counseling. Henry's presentation of a case, entitled "Anger in a Spiritual Sandpit," challenges all of us with a core experience that often arises with pain, or confusion, or disability. How we confront this experience matters. The counselor's simple, faithful presence in the moment to the pain of another invites us all to ask, "What would I do?" In addition, his reflections on various contraindications to incorporating spiritual elements into counseling are well worth pondering. In Chapter 12 we see Elliott Ingersoll's bold subtitle, "The Dance of Magic and Effort" come to life in his own spiritual journey and in the case of Jan, who struggles with a loving God and a painful world. Elliott's deep grounding in his own journey, spiritual practice, and learning is a testament of self-awareness for those attempting to integrate spirituality into practice. It makes a good final chapter, then, since it helps to summarize some important elements stated earlier.

The counselor's own pursuit of openness to a variety of traditions, as well as his or her devotion to a sustained spiritual practice, are critical elements that undergird the integration of spirituality into professional counseling. The lynchpin here is, as Elliott sees it, that the person of the counselor is the primary element in the process of integration.

All together, the twelve chapters of this book present a practical anthology of approaches to integrating spirituality into professional counseling practice. As a counselor educator, I am encouraged by my own students' reception of earlier drafts of this work. These chapters have stimulated class discussion about a range of topics including counselor identity, counselors' own self-awareness as well as their personal and professional development (sometimes called "self/person of the therapist" work), ethical ways to incorporate spiritual practices into counseling work, curiosity about different spiritual traditions and the need for "otherness experiences," development of one's own spiritual practice and learning about the skills needed to pass them on to others, and so on. I am pleased that these chapters function well as a platform from which students' own explorations can begin. This book can, I believe, serve as a useful starting point for a variety of readers.

### Acknowledgements

This is my fourth edited book. Over the years I have learned that when one sets out to pull together a book such as this, the process itself is a humbling task and the persons who assist in it deserve all the gratitude.

I am grateful, in the first place, to the ten contributors to this project. They shared generously of themselves and we are the better for it. Thank you.

I am grateful to Barry Fetterolf, Mary Falcon, and Lahaska Press for believing in this project. In these days, commitment of the necessary resources to bringing a publication to completion is not a small task, and it requires a certain level of trust (and some risk) in the writer/editor. I am grateful for their confidence. I also thank the reviewers who gave us very helpful advice on how to improve the first draft of the manuscript:

Timothy L. Barber, Cincinnati Christian University
James R. Beck, Denver Seminary
Karin Jordan, George Fox University
Robert H. Pate, Jr., University of Virginia
Patricia Stevens, Morehead State University
David Tobin, Gannon University

My colleagues in the Department of Counseling and Human Services at the University of Scranton have been both supportive and encouraging. My colleague, Liz Jacob, has been a supportive advisor throughout this project; I am grateful for her help and encouragement. My graduate assistants, Marlee Lemoncelli and Chris Whitney, have been wonderful and good-humored assistants, especially with procuring materials, word processing, tracking down publications, editing, and providing enthusiasm when needed.

As always, my wife, Ellen, has been a source of inspiration. One of the best natural counselors I have ever known, she weaves her own depth of soul and prayerful gentleness—along with a large measure of ability to challenge people to be their absolute best—into very competent clinical practice. And I should know. On many days I have needed these assets of hers in my own life! She is a gift of God to me. I am forever grateful.

I hope that the readers of this book will find it useful. It is intended to benefit graduate students in the fields of counseling and psychotherapy, as well as a wide range of helping professionals, psychotherapists, and professional counselors for whom the topic sparks interest. I know first-hand that attempting to integrate spiritual issues, sensitivities, and concerns within professional clinical practice is a daunting and rewarding task. I have learned the most about this work by listening to others who attempt it and are willing to tell the story. I hope this book provides the reader with a similar kind of learning.

## References

Abels, S. L. (2000). *Spirituality in social work practice: Narratives for professional helping.* Denver, CO: Love Publishing.

Barnum, B. S. (2003). *Spirituality in nursing: From traditional to new age.* New York, NY: Springer.

Becvar, D. (1994, August). Can spiritual yearnings and therapeutic goals be melded? *Family Therapy News,* pp. 13–14.

Bergin, A. E. (1991). Values and religious issues in psychotherapy and mental health. *American Psychologist, 46,* 394–403.

Bergin, A. E. (1980). Psychotherapy and religious values. *Journal of Consulting and Clinical Psychology, 48,* 75–105.

Borysenko, J. (1993). *Fire in the soul: A new psychology of spiritual optimism.* New York, NY: Warner.

Browning, D. S. (1987). *Religious thought and the modern psychologies: A critical conversation in the theology of culture.* Philadelphia, PA: Fortress.

Burke, M. T. (1998, Winter). From the Chair. *CACREP Connection, 2.*

Burke, M. T. & Miranti, J. G. (1992). *Ethical and spiritual values in counseling.* Alexandria, VA: American Counseling Association.

Burke, M. T. & Miranti, J. G. (1995). (Eds.). *Counseling: The spiritual dimension.* Alexandria, VA: American Counseling Association.

Burke, M. T., Chauvin, J. C., & Miranti, J. (*in press*). *Spirituality in counseling and therapy: A developmental and multicultural approach.* New York, NY: Brunner-Toutledge.

Council for Accreditation of Counseling and Related Educational Programs (CACREP). (2001). *CACREP accreditation manual.* Alexandria, VA: Author.

Canda, E. R. (1998). *Spirituality in social work: New directions.* New York, NY: Haworth Pastoral Press.

Canda, E. R. & Smith, E. D. (2001). *Transpersonal perspectives on spirituality in social work.* New York, NY: Haworth Press.

Chandler, C. K., Holden, J. M., & Kolander, C. A. (1992). Counseling for spiritual wellness: Theory and practice. *Journal of Counseling & Development, 71,* 168–175.

Clinebell, H .J. (1998). *Understanding and counseling persons with alcohol, drug, and behavioral addictions.: Counseling for recovery and prevention through psychology and religion* (rev.). Nashville, TN: Abingdon.

Frame, M. W. (2003). *Integrating religion and spirituality into counseling: A comprehensive approach.* Pacific Grove, CA: Brooks Cole.

Frame, M. W. (2000). The spiritual genogram in family therapy. *Journal of Marital and Family Therapy, 26*(2), 211–216.

Fukuyama, M. A. & Sevig, T. D. (1999). *Integrating spirituality into multicultural counseling.* Thousand Oaks: Sage.

Gaventa, W. C. & Coulter, D. L. (2002). *Spirituality and intellectual disability: International perspectives on the effect of culture and religion on healing body, mind and soul.* Binghamton, NY: Haworth.

Hackney, H. (2000). *Practice issues for the beginning counselor.* Needham Heights, MA: Allyn & Bacon.

Ingersoll, R.E. (1997). Teaching a course on counseling and spirituality. *Counseling and Values, 36,* 224–232.

Kelly, E. W. (1995). *Spirituality and religion in counseling and psychotherapy: Diversity in theory and practice.* Alexandria, VA: American Counseling Association.

Koenig, H. G. (1990). Research on religion and mental health in later life: A review and commentary. *Journal of Geriatric Psychiatry, 23,* 23–53.

Koenig, H .G. (2002). *Spirituality in patient care: Why, how, when, and what?*. Templeton Foundation Press.

Jonas, W. B. & Levin, J. S. (1999). *Essentials of complementary and alternative medicine*. Lippincott, Williams & Wilson.

Jordan, M. R. (1999). *Reclaiming your story: Family history and spiritual growth*. Westminster John Knox.

Larson, D. B., Lu, F. G., & Swyers, J. P. (1997). *Model curriculum for psychiatric residency training programs: Religion and spirituality in clinical practice, a course outline*. Rockville, MD: National Institute for Healthcare Research.

Levin, J. (2002). *God, faith, and health: Exploring the spirituality-healing connection*. New York, NY: Wiley.

Miller, W. R. (1999). (Ed.). *Integrating spirituality into treatment: Resources for practitioners*. Washington, DC: American Psychological Association.

Morgan, O. J. (1987). Pastoral counseling and petitionary prayer. *Journal of Religion and Health, 26*(2), 149–152.

Morgan, O. J. (1989). Elements in a spirituality of pastoral care. *The Journal of Pastoral Care, 43*, 99–109.

Morgan, O. J. (2000). "Counseling and spirituality." In H. C. Hackney (Ed.), *Practice issues for the beginning counselor* (pp. 170–182). Needham Heights, MA: Allyn & Bacon.

Morgan, O. J. (2002a). Spirituality, alcohol and other drug problems: Where have we been? Where are we going? *Alcoholism Treatment Quarterly, 20*(3/4), 61–82.

Morgan, O. J. (2002b). Alcohol problems, alcoholism and spirituality: An overview of measurement and scales. *Alcoholism Treatment Quarterly, 20*(1), 1–18.

Morgan, O. J. & Jordan, M. (Eds.). (1999). *Addiction and spirituality: A multidisciplinary approach*. St. Louis, MO: Chalice.

Pargament, K. I. (1997). *The psychology of religion and coping: Theory, research, practice*. New York: Guilford.

Richards, P. S. and Bergin, A. E. (1997). *A spiritual strategy for counseling and psychotherapy*. Washington, DC: American Psychological Association.

Ringwald, C. D. (2002). *The soul of recovery: Uncovering the spiritual dimension in the treatment of addictions*. New York, NY: Oxford University Press.

Shafranske, E. P. (1996). (Ed.). *Religion and the clinical practice of psychology*. Washington, DC: American Psychological Association.

Shea, J. (2000). *Spirituality & health care: Reaching toward a holistic future*. Chicago, IL: Park Ridge Center.

Shelly, J. A. (2000). *Spiritual care: A guide for caregivers*. Downers Grove, IL: InterVarsity Press.

Stanard, R. P., Sandhu, D. S., & Painter, L. C. (2000). Assessment of spirituality in counseling. *Journal of Counseling & Development, 78*, 204–210.

Steere, D. A. (1997). *Spiritual presence in psychotherapy: A guide for care givers*. New York, NY: Brunner/Mazel.

Sue, D. W., Arredondo, P. & McDavis, R .J. (1992). Multicultural counseling competencies and standards: A call to the profession. *Journal of Counseling & Development, 70*, 477–486.

Taylor, E .J. (2001). *Spiritual care: Nursing theory, research, and practice.* New York, NY: Prentice Hall.

VandeCreek, L. (1999). (Ed.). *Spiritual care for persons with dementia: Fundamental for pastoral practice.* Binghamton, NY: Haworth.

Vash, C. L. (1994). *Personality and adversity: Psychospiritual aspects of rehabilitation.* New York, NY: Springer.

Vash, C. L. & McCarthy, H. (1995). Spirituality, disability and rehabilitation. Special double issue of *Rehabilitation Education, 9* (2 & 3), 1995.

Walsh, F. (1999). *Spiritual resources in family therapy.* New York, NY: Guilford.

Witmer, J. M. & Sweeney, T. J. (1992). A holistic model for wellness and prevention over the life span. *Journal of Counseling & Development, 71,* 140–149.

# About the Contributors

### Clifford Brooks, Ph.D.

"Ford" is an associate professor in the Department of Counseling at Shippensburg University (PA). He received his doctorate and educational specialist degrees in counseling from the College of William and Mary and his master's degree from Virginia Commonwealth University in Rehabilitation Counseling. Ford is a Licensed Professional Counselor (LPC), a Nationally Certified Counselor (NCC), and a Certified Addiction Counselor (CAC). He currently is on the Board of Directors of the Center for Credentialing and Education, Inc. (CCE). Ford presents regionally, nationally, and internationally on spirituality and addiction issues, focusing much of his writing in these areas.

Ford is an avid runner, nature enthusiast, juggler, and magician. He and his wife Kathryn, along with their daughter Sarah, reside in Shippensburg, Pennsylvania.

### Mary Alice Bruce, Ph.D.

Mary Alice, formerly a mathematics teacher and professional school counselor, is currently an associate professor who coordinates the school counseling program at the University of Wyoming. Mary Alice is a Licensed Professional Counselor (LPC), a Nationally Certified Counselor (NCC), and Certified K–12 Professional School Counselor. Currently, she is a member of the CACREP 2008 Standards Revision Committee and Co-Chair of the ACA International Committee.

Yoga as well as cross country skiing and snowshoeing in the Rocky Mountains with her husband, children, family, and friends offer fun times to complement her work with children and adolescents.

### Craig S. Cashwell, Ph.D.

Craig is Professor and Director of Graduate Studies in the Department of Counseling and Educational Development at the University of North Carolina at Greensboro. He earned his Ph.D. in Counselor Education from the University of North Carolina at Greensboro and taught for six years at Mississippi State University prior to returning home to teach at UNCG. Craig is a Licensed Professional Counselor (LPC), Nationally Certified Counselor (NCC), Approved Clinical Supervisor (ACS), and a Certified Breath Therapy Facilitator. He is the co-editor of *Integrating Religion and Spirituality in Counseling: A Guide to Competent Practice,* published by the American Counseling Association in 2005.

When not engaged in academic pursuits, Craig can be found with his wife, Dr. Tammy Cashwell, and Samantha, their daughter, his daily reminders of the joy and bliss in laughter, love, and life. Craig wishes to dedicate his chapter to the memory of his late father, Jerry J. Cashwell, who remains his greatest teacher.

### Mary A. Fukuyama, Ph.D.

Mary received her Ph.D. from Washington State University and has worked at the University of Florida Counseling Center for the past twenty-three years as a counseling psychologist, supervisor and trainer. She is a clinical professor and teaches courses on spirituality and multicultural counseling for the Department of Counselor Education and also the Counseling Psychology Program. She co-authored with Todd Sevig, *Integrating Spirituality into Multicultural Counseling.* She was recently recognized as a Fellow by Division 17 (Counseling Psychology) of the American Psychological Association. Her practice specialties include multicultural counseling, working with university students from a developmental perspective, and counselor training.

She is an active member of the University of Florida's Center for Spirituality and Health and her current research interests include conducting a qualitative study on "multicultural expressions" of spirituality. Her leisure interests include birding, kayaking, music, and art.

### Michael Tlanusta Garrett, Ph.D.

Michael, Eastern Band of Cherokee, is Professor of Counseling and Chair of the Department of Educational Leadership and Counseling at Old Dominion University (VA). He holds a Ph.D. in Counseling and Counselor Education and a M.Ed. in Counseling and Development from the University of North Carolina at Greensboro. Author and co-author of more than fifty articles and chapters dealing with multiculturalism, group work, wellness and spirituality, school counseling, working with youth, and counseling Native Americans, Michael has also authored the book, *Walking on the Wind: Cherokee Teachings for Harmony and Balance* (1998). His most recent co-authored book is *Native American Faith in America* (2003).

Michael has worked as a school counselor at the middle and high school levels, as a college student personnel worker with Native American and other minority students in the university setting, as an individual and group therapist in a family services agency setting, and as a project director in an urban Native American center serving the local Native American community. Michael grew up on the Cherokee Indian reservation in the mountains of western North Carolina. Currently, he lives in Chesapeake, Virginia with his wife, Claudia, and his son, Gavin.

### R. Elliott Ingersoll, Ph.D.

Elliott is currently a professor and the chairperson of the department of Counseling, Administration, Supervision, & Adult Learning in the College of Education and Human Services at Cleveland State University. He is a licensed psychologist and clinical counselor in the state of Ohio where his areas of specialization are mood disorders, anxiety disorders, religious and spiritual problems, and substance abuse.

Elliott is author or co-author of four books and over two dozen journal articles and book chapters. His areas of publication are psychopharmacology, spirituality, and applying Ken Wilber's integral theory. He has studied and practiced contemplative techniques from Christian traditions, Kripalu Yoga, as well as Earth-based religions. He lives in Kent, Ohio, with his wife, Jennifer; son, Brady; and daughter Kaitlyn.

### Henry McCarthy, Ph.D.

Henry has worked in the field of rehabilitation since the 1970s. He earned a Ph.D. with a specialization in rehabilitation from the Psychology Department at the University of Kansas. From there he completed a postdoctoral fellowship at the Rusk Institute of Rehabilitation Medicine in New York and became Director of Psychosocial Research (NIDRR-funded) at the Human Resources Center. For the past twenty years he has taught and supervised students pursuing careers in rehabilitation counseling at the Louisiana State University Health Sciences Center.

The primary thrust of Henry's professional work has been to promote genuine collaboration and advocacy among the disability, rehabilitation, and employment communities. His service to the profession includes being the current Associate Editor of *Rehabilitation Counseling Bulletin* and the former Associate Editor of *Rehabilitation Education*. World cultures and travel are his main avocation, along with swimming and playing tennis. He resides in New Orleans with his wonderful wife and two teenage sons.

## Oliver Morgan, Ph.D.

Ollie is Professor and Chair of the Department of Counseling and Human Services at the University of Scranton (PA). He earned his Ph.D. in pastoral psychotherapy from Boston University and holds masters degrees in both Marriage & Family Therapy, and Divinity. He is a Nationally Certified Counselor (NCC), a Licensed Marital & Family Therapist (LMFT) in Pennsylvania, and an Approved Clinical Supervisor (ACS).

When not teaching or pursuing research, he can be found reading Civil War history, listening to jazz music, and spending time with his wife, Ellen, and their three children: Sierra, Danny, and Rusty. The simple pleasures of seeing the world fresh through their eyes and sharing those moments with Ellen is the great blessing of his life.

## Daya Singh Sandhu, Ed.D.

Daya is Professor and Chair of the Department of Educational & Counseling Psychology at University of Louisville in Kentucky. He has authored or edited several books, numerous book chapters, and more than 50 articles in refereed journals. Some of Daya's books include, *Counseling for Prejudice Prevention and Reduction* (1997); *Violence in American Schools: A Practical Guide for Counselors* (2000); *Faces of Violence: Psychological Correlates, Concepts, and Intervention Strategies* (2001); and *Elementary School Counseling in the New Millennium* (2001).

Daya was recently honored as one of the twelve pioneers in multicultural counseling. Sage published his autobiographical account in the *Handbook of Multicultural Counseling* (2001) (second edition). In addition, he is a recipient of the AMCD Multicultural Research Award (2000) and, in 2001, received a Fulbright Research Award for India to conduct cross-cultural studies on depression.

## Rebecca Powell Stanard, Ph.D.

Rebecca is an associate professor in Counseling and Educational Psychology at the University of West Georgia in Carrollton, Georgia. She is a graduate of Ohio University and has experience as a counselor in a wide variety of settings. Rebecca has served as an editorial board member for several professional journals and is currently vice chair of the board of directors for the Council for Accreditation of Counseling and Related Education Programs (CACREP). Her research interests include spirituality in counseling and counselor education and effective teaching and supervision methods.

Her personal interests include reading, photography, and traveling. Her two passions are teaching and baseball, not necessarily in that order. She also suffers from delusions of efficacy as a home improvement guru. Perhaps her most notable accomplishment is that she is the mother of two grown sons, Mark and David, who are remarkable human beings. She lives a joy-filled life with her companion and their four cats.

**Richard Watts, Ph.D.**

Richard is Professor and Director of the Ph.D. program in Counselor Education at Sam Houston State University in Huntsville, TX. He has published over sixty journal articles and book chapters and five books. Richard serves as editorial board member for several professional journals and is a member of the board of directors for the Council for Accreditation of Counseling and Related Educational Programs (CACREP). His professional and research interests include Adlerian, cognitive, and constructivist approaches to individual, group, and couple and family counseling; counselor supervision and counselor efficacy; ethical and legal issues; play therapy; and religions and spiritual issues in counseling.

His hobbies include playing guitar and piano, reading, and spending time with his family. He lives with his two favorite people in the world: Cheryl, his wife of twenty-five years, and Will, his five-year-old son.

❧

# CHAPTER ONE

# Counseling's Fifth Force

## Oliver J. Morgan

> If you attend the soul closely enough, with an educated and
> steadfast imagination, changes take place without your being
> aware of them until they are all over and well in place.
>
> —Moore, 1992, p. 19

Thomas Moore, contemporary psychotherapist and spiritual guide, speaks eloquently of the need to reimagine the clinical disciplines, so that attention to spiritual issues, values, concerns, and practices can be integrated into their view. He advocates for more attention to care of the soul as a complementary attitude and approach to the cure of mental and emotional problems in living (Moore, 1992). While many have begun to address this challenge in the years since it was first offered, much work still remains to integrate spirituality fully into counseling and psychotherapy.

There is now a growing interest in spirituality within the clinical disciplines. A recent consensus report, produced by teams of scholars from a range of clinical disciplines, illustrates this growing attention. Sponsored by the National Institute for Healthcare Research (NIHR) and funded by The John Templeton Foundation, these working groups set out to study "the quality as well as the *state-of-the-science* of the literature in religion and spirituality as it relates to clinical health status" (Larson, Swyers & McCullough, 1997, p. 7; *italics mine*). These well-respected teams of researchers represented a variety of clinical disciplines including psychology, psychiatry, sociology, primary care medicine, epidemiology,

1

research design, alcohol and drug abuse treatment and prevention, public health, and the neurosciences. The title of their published work is *Scientific Research on Spirituality and Health: A Consensus Report* (1997). Forty years ago, such an endeavor, and certainly the title and stated purpose of such an investigation, would have been unthinkable. As Sandra Schneiders (1990) notes, in scientific and educated circles the term *spirituality* once connoted mindless piety or subjectivism; now it is used to suggest deeper elements of human life and activity. We have come a fair distance from those earlier days. The careful and critical, although highly positive, attention these scholars and practitioners give to spirituality in their consensus report is all the more compelling because of its "best science" approach.

## What Do You Mean, "Spirituality"?

Spirituality, from the Latin word *spiritus,* meaning "breath," is a fundamental orientation to one's life and to the ground of all life; it is the source of one's posture toward living, of the nature of one's connection to all things, and of one's perception of an ultimate reality. One's spirituality engenders a way of being and experiencing, involving meaning, wholeness, openness to the infinite, and connectedness to others and the natural world (Kurtz, 1999; ASERVIC White Paper, 1997); it eventuates in specific behaviors. Anne Carr says it well: "Spirituality is expressed in everything one does. On the individual level, it is a style, unique to the self, that catches up all one's attitudes . . . in behavior, bodily expressions, life choices, in what one supports and affirms, and what one protests and denies. . . . [It] is deeply informed by family, teachers, friends, community, class, race, culture, sex, and by one's time in history, just as it is influenced by personal beliefs, intellectual positions, and moral options" (1988, pp. 202–203).

It is important to distinguish between spirituality and religion. Again, Carr (1988), speaking as a professional theologian, says it succinctly: "spirituality can be understood as the source of both theology and morality. For it is the experience out of which both derive as a human response" (1988, p. 202). As Thomas Hart says, "in relation to organized religion, spirituality is both prior and more personal; it is the reason religious organizations come into being" (Hart, 2002, p. 23). One may see spirituality as the essential inner core of all religions, the essence toward which all the doctrines, symbols, and religious rituals points, the experience sine qua non that religion is supposed to facilitate. It is understood to be both the wellspring and goal of religious practice.

Commonly accepted definitions or descriptions of religion include notions such as "a medium of organized worship and fellowship" and "the expression of beliefs in conduct and ritual" (Ingersoll, 1995, p. 11). Rooted in the Latin word *religio,* "a binding together," religion is related to practices and beliefs that bind human beings to the divine and to one another. Religions are integrated expressions of beliefs and doctrines that are made concrete in rituals, symbols, social identity, lifestyles, conduct, and often institutions with organizing elements such as hierarchies or elders. Religions may be seen as a "variety of frameworks through which spirituality is expressed" (Ingersoll, 1995, p. 12). In the context of religion, spirituality may be understood as a "lived theology" (Kurtz, 1999, p. 20), a set of perceptions, experiences, and beliefs that result in a way of living.

Clearly, the current interest in spirituality is occurring among many people, and it is not confined to churchgoers or to publicly identified religious people. It is widespread and inquisitive. However, I believe that we are not at a place where we can fully define spirituality with any real confidence. Not yet! Many publications attempt such definitions, and, as with many of life's most important issues, the definitions never quite seem to hit the mark. Let me suggest a place to begin. We've discussed how spirituality and religion are different. Let's look briefly at how they intersect.

We alluded earlier to the consensus report from the National Institute for Healthcare Research (Larson, Swyers & McCullough, 1997) entitled, *Scientific Research on Spirituality and Health.* The NIHR panels began with a view of *both* spirituality and religion as multidimensional, complex phenomena, and attempted to describe their fundamental characteristics in relationship to health. Rather than beginning theoretically and abstractly, they focused pragmatically. By moving to practical application within health-related areas, they could focus on similarities and mutual contributions.

The panels began with empirical studies that suggested that as many as 74 percent of people surveyed see themselves as both religious *and* spiritual. Reversing a trend toward seeing spirituality primarily as something independent of religion, and thus as something different from what many people experience in their lives, the panels attempt to provide some sense of the *overlap* in these two phenomena. They believe that this can facilitate a focus on multidimensional data useful for understanding the contributions of each to pragmatic healing and health.

The panels identified a "primary criterion" and "common denominator" for both spirituality and religion:

> Both spirituality and religion involve the subjective feelings, thoughts, and behaviors that arise from a search for the sacred. The term "search" refers to attempts to identify, articulate, maintain, or transform. The term "sacred" refers to a divine being or Ultimate Reality or Ultimate Truth as perceived by the individual.    (Larson, Swyers & McCullough 1997, p. 22)

Thus, the central focus on the *sacred* for both spirituality and religion is affirmed in this report. While each individual's and group's notion of the sacred is socially and culturally influenced, it stands nevertheless as *that which attracts one's devotion and commitment,* as *the divine or ultimate in one's life.* There is also a critical element of *search* as a criterion. The *attempt to identify what is sacred, the ability to articulate it somehow, to maintain contact with it, and enter into transformation in the face of it* are all parts of the search process.

The central elements here are the *sacred* and a process of *search* that is cognitive, emotional, behavioral, and experiential. Although many individuals "approach the sacred through the personal, subjective, and experiential path of spirituality; it is also apparent that this experiential path often includes organizational or institutional beliefs and practices [religious in nature]" (Larson, Swyers & McCullough, 1997, p. 17).

Spirituality, as a search for the sacred, is about discovering the fundamental roots of existence, the meaning of living, or discovering what is worthy of one's full devotion and commitment. Religion may provide companionship, nourishment, guidelines, and outlets for the spiritual quest; it provides community for spiritual seekers and spiritual traditions within which seekers can situate themselves.

Spirituality need not be discussed in supernatural terms or with religious language. It may be understood in more *humanistic* ways, using the language of philosophy and anthropology such as self-transcendence, connectedness, reverence for life, ultimate meaning. It may be an experience of nature, of connection with others, of a horizon toward which one strives, and the deep experiences that give human life meaning, such as the birth of a child, or the blessedness of nature. Then again, spirituality may be nourished by a language that is more *religious and theological,* that speaks of being "made in the image and likeness of God," of God's gracious activity in the world, of creation and the Creator that gives it meaning and worth, of searching *and* being found. Here, the experience is described more often as the relationship with a personal being and a lifestyle based on following the will of God.

For the purposes of this book, whether one conceptualizes spirituality in its more humanistic or its more theistic ways, the common denominators of *search* and *sacredness* still apply.

## How Did We Get Here?

The goal of spirituality is the alleviation of mental, emotional, and spiritual distress thought to be at least in part caused by the lack of an appropriate relationship with ultimate reality, most often signaled by and reflected in inappropriate relationships with other people and things. Spirituality is less a method than an attitude, a posture of one's very being that allows seeing not different things but everything differently. . . .     (Kurtz, 1999, p. 20)

Why the current interest in spirituality within the counseling and clinical worlds? Spirituality has been described recently as "the quintessential element of the human condition," a universal and "intimate part of the human condition" (Cornett, 1998, pp. 157–158). This is strong language that would have seemed quaint, or odd, or even dangerous only thirty years ago! While the notion of integrating a spiritual vision and set of values into the task of human healing and health is an old one, it has gone through a number of changes over time, particularly in the United States.

In recent years, a number of scholars in the clinical disciplines have proposed an outline of historical and cultural developments that have led to this point (Benner, 1988; Browning, 1987; Holifield, 1983; Kurtz, 1999; McNeill, 1951; Oden, 1984; Rieff, 1966; Steere, 1997; Torrey, 1986). Although I cannot do justice to the depth and insight of these historical and cultural studies in the space available, I present a picture of developments that set the stage for the current rise of interest in spirituality and try to provide a context for the current book.[1]

---

[1] The historical examination below is highly selective and painted with broad strokes. It reflects some of my interests and experiences as a Christian, a recovering person, and a professional counselor and educator. Others would no doubt add or highlight different events, persons, and themes to this historical picture and thereby would enhance its inclusivity. I invite the reader to do so. I believe, however, that the major point here remains valid, namely that authentic care of persons has always had roots in concern for the *whole* person. In providing such care, understanding the need to include spiritual beliefs and values has ebbed and flowed. As we move into the twenty-first century, the opportunity for true integration of spirituality into the care of persons has become an important task.

The roots of psychology as a profession and as a discipline lie deep in spiritual soil. The etymological root *psyche* is the classic Greek concept of soul. Psychology is literally the study of the soul, the very essence of what it is to be human. Long before there were psychologists, people brought their psychic troubles to their spiritual leaders. Many still do.         (Miller & Delaney, 2005, p. 291)

Modern counseling and psychotherapy are descendents of a long and proud tradition of soul care. This tradition was part and parcel of early Western philosophy and the Judeo-Christian religious traditions. The pursuit of perennial truths and right living was honored as the work that led to healing and wellness. Philosophers, wise guides, rabbis, gurus, and pastors saw themselves as facilitators of that work. They were the counselors of their day, and their part in the healing task was well understood.

These counselors tended the "soul." The Greek words *psyche* (soul) and *pneuma* (spirit), the Hebrew *ruach* (breath of life), all refer to the "life force" or essence of the whole person, the central unifying element of human body, mind, and spirit. The seat of this element was conceived of as the soul (Miller & Delaney, 2005).

Across the expanse of history and a variety of cultures, approaches to soul care had common elements and utilized the tools of philosophy, religion, or person-to-person healing. Living rightly and in harmony with the divine and other persons was understood to bring peace and health. Illness was (and is often still today!) seen as a "symbolic expression of internal conflicts" and dis-ease within the whole person or as the result of "disturbed relations with others" (Frank, 1963, pp. 49–50). Soul care, then, has been understood as nourishing and supporting right relations with others and guiding individuals to come to terms with internal and relational difficulties.

Plato and Socrates described themselves as "physicians/healers of the soul," believing that philosophy could help to lead persons toward perfection and right living, the "good life" (Benner, 1988). Zeno and Plutarch provided lists of virtues that would guide the learner in living, and offered personal models of the good life, who were to be emulated (Kurtz, 1999). Wise men and prophets in ancient Israel helped the people to live justly and "walk humbly with their God" (Micah 6:8). Confessors, pastors, desert guides, and spiritual directors in early Christianity served a similar purpose, counseling others on personal conduct, just living, and their relationships to God and others.

Both in earlier times and today, Islam's *Koran* and the five *Pillars* as well as the guidance offered by imams and ayatollahs; Hinduism's

*Bhagavad Gita* and *Upanishads,* offering advice on spiritual truths and ways of living them out; Buddhism's *Four Noble Truths* and *Eightfold Path,* as well as the models and guidance from monks and Zen Masters— all these and other religious traditions offer holistic and spiritual ways of understanding the world and living rightly within it.

This chapter presents a point of view that sees the modern psychologies as descendents of religious and spiritual traditions of care. Browning (1987) makes the point that one can also see the religious and philosophical traditions of care as "ancient psychologies" with "psychotherapeutic implications" (p. 4). His book cogently lays out the mutual "horizons" shared by both religious and spiritual traditions of care and the modern psychologies, even when they are unaware of the common ground. These disciplines and approaches are in many important ways "soul mates."

Of course, many other cultures have always had, and continue to have, their guides for living rightly, for nurturing a spiritual life, and caring holistically for their people. These natural healers (*curanderas,* witch-doctors, *manangs,* and so forth) abound in many parts of the globe (Kurtz, 1999; Torrey, 1986).[2] And it is important to note that, while there is great diversity in healing practices and designated healers around the world, there are similarities across cultural traditions (Frank, 1963).

In the United States and Western Europe, well into the eighteenth and nineteenth centuries, there was a variety of healers and guides for human care and development of soul: priests, rabbis, shamans, pastors, and the like. There was a consensus on the form and goal of soul work. There were many healers who brought to their craft a vision of human persons, embedded within creation and the natural world, as well as interconnected within a social milieu; these natural healers encouraged behavior that mirrored and fostered this sense of connectedness and compassion.

Their spiritual vision, and the counseling that conveyed it, sometimes had a supernatural ground, but not always. The vision promoted by a variety of healers and guides sought to be transformative and healing, but was not always oriented explicitly to theological concepts of salvation. Religion, theology, and philosophy were the natural allies of this vision, but its lifeblood was belief in a common humanity and a lifestyle that was rooted in compassion and connection. Soul care in all its forms sought to nourish this vision and lifestyle as a healthful way of life.

---

[2]I have found the work of Harvard psychiatrist Arthur Kleinman (1980, 1988, 1989) very helpful in exploring the common cultural elements among healers and among the processes of healing around the world.

The rise of science and secularization brought with it much promise and a tendency to fill in the gaps in human understanding. The movement toward a more secular psychology and psychotherapy as primary forms of soul care was aided by the development of modern science in the eighteenth and nineteenth centuries, and the development of a scientific psychology in the late nineteenth and early twentieth centuries. These developments of the modern period are indeed great human achievements, and they have brought unparalleled benefits to the modern world. However, another result of these developments was the decline of religion's intellectual respectability and a spiritual void left by its demise (Benner, 1988).

In this new, modern world, the psychotherapist replaced the spiritual guide or pastor as healer of souls and advisor for right living. And he or she performed these functions from within a vision of reality denuded of any religious faith, of any sense of the sacred, or of centuries-old traditions of the good life.

Increasingly, the care of souls became more of a pastoral function, as religious sensibilities became more focused in churches and congregations. However, the care and health of humans, their psyches and behavior, increasingly became the domain of medicine and science, led by psychology and psychoanalysis, and beholden to a succession of seemingly transformative mantras like self-acceptance, self-actualization, self-realization, or adjustment (Holifield, 1983).

While religion often abandoned the task of dialogue with science and retreated within its sanctuaries, psychology and science all too often ignored religion and "all its works and pomps," or treated them as misguided and even dangerous. As Kurtz (1999) has stated the case, both psychotherapy and religion/spirituality came to know each other "mainly by caricature" (p. 31). At the beginning of the nineteenth century, evangelical revivalism and poetic romanticism railed against this "invasion" of the human arena by science and increasing secularity at every level, but they were powerless to stop its advance (Holifield, 1983).

## A Form of Protest and a Way Forward

Yet, early in twentieth-century America, there were attempts to reconcile these divisions.[3] Some of these were more humanistic, others more theological or religious. These were ways of opening dialogue and collaboration

---

[3] I am indebted to the work of Ernest Kurtz (1979 & 1999) and E. Brooks Holifield (1983) for much of the substance in the discussion of this period that follows.

between more scientific and psychological approaches and ways of proceeding that were more religious and spiritually sensitive.

There were important movements like (a) the *Emmanuel Movement,* an effort to integrate theology with therapy, with ties to the mainstream medical establishment of its day; (b) the advent of the *mental hygiene movement* and the work of Clifford Beers, one of the early forbears of professional counseling; (c) the *pastoral care movement,* led by Anton Boisen, and symbolized by the rise of pastoral counseling and clinical-pastoral education; and (d) the birth of a new scholarly field of inquiry called the *psychology of religion,* which explored the potential of religious experience to nourish personality development, or move a person "from egoism to altruism" (Wulff, 1996 & 1997; Holifield, 1983, p. 199). All these movements advocated dialogue and cooperation between scientific and spiritual/religious perspectives.

There were also important thinkers and writers in earlier decades of the twentieth century who advocated mutual attention between psychotherapy and religion, and who laid groundwork for the rise of interest in spirituality. We've already mentioned Anton Boisen, whose autobiographical and theological works *Out of the Depths* (1960) and *The Exploration of the Inner World* (1936) were influential in the beginnings of the clinical-pastoral training of ministers, and Clifford Beers, whose autobiography, *A Mind That Found Itself* (1944), was a scathing critique of the mental health system of his day and the catalyst for the mental hygiene movement, which was seen as a way to unite religion and health. With credentials and colleagues in both the clinical and religious worlds, these thinkers and prodigious writers influenced the conversation between those disciplines.

There were also critically important writers of the time from the fields of the psychology of religion, such as William James in *The Varieties of Religious Experience* (1902) and Rollo May in *The Art of Counseling* (1939), and from clinical-pastoral education, such as Richard Cabot and his work in training for ministry (Cabot, 1908; Cabot & Dicks, 1936), who were making important contributions. Again, they possessed credentials as men of science who regarded the whole person—including areas of religion and spirituality—with respect. They helped to bring a thaw in previously chilly relations between these fields of inquiry.

And there was the ongoing protest against one-sided secular views of health and humanity made by the emerging Twelve Step programs (such as Alcoholics Anonymous) and their success with previously intractable problems, rooted in a view of human health that integrated spiritual concerns (Morgan, 2002). Begun in the mid-1930s, AA and the Twelve Step movement had a powerful impact on those physicians, scientists, and pastors who were associated with it, as well as on the popular media of the day. The AA view of alcoholism and addiction as a "three-fold disease"—that is, physical, psychological, and spiritual—has evolved over time into an important contribution to the current more holistic view of illness in general (Morgan, 1999; Morgan & Jordan, 1999). The influence of the Twelve Step spiritual view is one of the cultural factors that is a catalyst for renewed interest in the topic for counselors and other clinical professionals today (see page 17, Influence of Group Movements, including Twelve Step Fellowships).

There were, of course, countervailing cultural developments and influences, particularly within the field of psychology, that opposed (or ignored) these developments and promoted a more secular view of human nature and a therapeutic role for psychology. Psychoanalysis, behaviorism, the "scientific psychologies," and psychiatry all fought to keep spirituality and religion separate from anything respectably clinical. Yet, each of these disciplines and the movements within traditional clinical care in the twentieth century have had their own rebels (think of C. G. Jung or Victor Frankl), who upheld a more integrative view of human living and its connections to the spiritual. Marsha Frame (2003, pp. 163–178, 218–232) has described these rebellions against secularizing elements in clinical care—which rebellions she calls "implicit approaches to religious and spiritual issues"—with amazing clarity. She also suggests a number of strategies for integrating spirituality and counseling that can be incorporated into a variety of counseling modalities (Frame, 2003, pp. 183–208, 232–235).

William Miller, in his fascinating study of "quantum change," or sudden personal transformations, in psychology (2001, p. 6), describes the "family resemblance" that pastoral counseling and the psychology of religion bear to the original unity of psychology and theology, of spirituality and clinical care. We have, I believe, come full circle in our understanding of the fundamental unity of human persons, a unity that is bio-psycho-social *and spiritual.* Now, as we move into the twenty-first century, we are in position to build on this rediscovered insight and bring a fully integrated approach to the care of persons.

I am a student of pastoral psychotherapy and counseling—specializing in the understanding and treatment of addictive disease. Learning about the historical roots and development of clinical care, as I have briefly traced it here, has been the crucible within which my own approach to integrating spirituality and counseling has been shaped and tested. I have learned from scholarship *and from my clients* about the value of a more integrated perspective that is open to spiritual experience and that works to move toward change in vision and behavior. I have also learned that our clients expect nothing less from us than an effort toward this integration.

## Components of Contemporary Interest in Spirituality

It is clear then that, as we begin our journey through the twenty-first century, the stage has been set for a resurgence of interest in spirituality as part of the human condition, and for a movement toward integrating spirituality into clinical care.

Signs of renewed interest in spirituality abound. In fiction, film, and the arts, spiritual topics are pursued with gusto and receive popular support; think of films such as *The Fisher King* or *The Passion of the Christ,* or the ongoing publishing success of M. Scott Peck's "road less traveled" book series (Peck, 1978, 1998a & b, 2003). The pursuit of spiritual retreats, wide examination of a variety of spiritual traditions (such as Eastern meditation and practices) by people in all walks of life, commitment to spirit- and faith-based social movements such as the Million-Man March and Promise Keepers or ecologically based care for the earth, the popularity and attendance at various conferences on spirituality and religion, even within mainstream science outlets—all these examples and more attest to the current cultural interest in spirituality (Myers, 2000). It is also clear that this cultural interest is mirrored in the expectations and desires of our clients in counseling and psychotherapy.

Where does this current interest come from? What are its sources? Scholars suggest a number of reasons for the rise of contemporary interest in spirituality. I wish to examine briefly a number of contemporary influences that, I believe, have given rise to the modern interest in spirituality.

- The advent of postmodern constructionism (Frame, 2003; Steere, 1997).

The "postmodern" approach privileges multiple perspectives and honors a variety of perceptions about the world over abstract, universal principles and fundamental absolutes. The construction of meaning, truth, and purpose emerges for persons in light of their relationships, language, culture, politics, and idiosyncratic experiences. And meaning *is* constructed; it is not handed down or discovered by those who search for it, as though it were something embedded in the objective fabric of things and waiting to be found. In the postmodern world, no dogma, either religious or psychological, holds ultimate sway or commands unswerving devotion. People construct the events and meanings of their lives subjectively, and live accordingly.

Clients' religious and spiritual beliefs are, then, part of the subjective reality they bring with them, and this reality is shaped by the communities of which they are a part. The job of clinical caregivers is to understand these beliefs and meanings, and to work within clients' realities.

• Increased attention to the outcomes of social science research into development of "healthy families," "wellness," and "spiritual well-being" (Ellison, 1983; Ingersoll, 1995; Larson, Swyers & McCullough, 1997).

Since the 1960s and 1970s, social science research has learned the value of inquiring into religious and spiritual variables as part of the investigation of health. The "quality of life" research that emerged out of the social indicators movement is a case in point (Moberg & Brusek, 1978). Significant weaknesses in the quality of life literature were seen to emerge from the neglect and sometimes complete omission of meaningful religious variables, due in large measure to the alienation of social science from religion and to the rigidity of methodological orthodoxy. Religion and spirituality were seen as improper, too difficult and unsuited to scientific investigation.

Sociological research into "spiritual well-being" (Moberg, 1967, 1971, 1986) as well as explorations into the "strengths" of healthy families (Stinnett & De Frain, 1985) were developed to address these weaknesses. These approaches also validated the power for good of spiritual wellness and/or religious values, commitments, and characteristics for individuals and families. As results such as these became more widely known, they encouraged a wider movement that asserted the role of spirituality in the public domain and in scientific investigation (Larson, Swyers & McCullough, 1997; Moberg, 1984; Paloutzian & Ellison, 1984).

• The contemporary emphasis on holistic thinking and movements to include supplemental and alternative medicine approaches (Frame, 2003; Steere, 1997).

As a bio-psycho-social paradigm of illness and health (Engel, 1980) has taken hold, coupled with deeper appreciation of ecological approaches to biological and social systems, more and more people have come to see the value of integrating the healing arts, psychotherapy, counseling, and spirituality (Chandler, Holden & Kolander, 1992; Witmer & Sweeney, 1992). The widely accepted 1940s and 1950s metaphor of the YMCA triangle of body, mind, and spirit—where there were distinct boundaries between each dimension and everyone (such as physicians, counselors, clergy) knew his or her place in the scheme of health—has given way to newer metaphors such as the wellness wheel (Witmer & Sweeney, 1992; Steere, 1997), or the turn to Native American models like the Way of the Circle (Garrett, 1996; Lake, 1991), or the balance found in connection to nature and the earth (Wilbur, 1999a & b).

In these newer perspectives, the boundaries are more fluid; multidisciplinary teams and processes are in vogue; and scientists and scholars are working in cross-disciplinary teams and exploring areas previously considered off-limits. Physical health and healing are now seen as more continuous with emotional, developmental, natural, and spiritual health. People in general more easily turn now to supplementing traditional medicine with such things as meditation, relaxation, nutrition, fitness, yoga, massage, acupuncture, bioenergetics, *ayurveda,* and reflexology. The list goes on (Steere, 1997). A variety of healing approaches are acceptable, and are seen to work in concert for maximum impact.

Some intriguing findings from the health Panels of NIHR (Larson, Swyers & McCullough, 1997) help explain this increasing interest:

• Patients with chronic medical illnesses (such as cystic fibrosis, diabetes, and various forms of cancer) frequently use religious and spiritual practices as adjuncts to medical care and report positive benefits.

• There appears to be a reduction in mortality in general for those who attend worship services more frequently, especially the elderly.

• Meditation is reported to have a number of positive health benefits, including lowering blood pressure, reducing chronic pain, increasing quality of life, and increasing longevity.

• Spirituality among cancer survivors is associated with positive health, reduced anxiety, and reduced levels of pain.

• Many religious beliefs and practices are associated with reduced involvement in illness-producing risky behaviors, for example, abusive drinking, smoking, and other drug use.

• New Age practices emphasize psychospiritual approaches that integrate traditional psychotherapies with spiritual awareness and practices, with the ultimate goal of personal growth and self-realization (Steere, 1997).

The holistic approach to health has had an effect on psychotherapy as well. It is much more common now—despite a long history of antagonism—to see traditional psychotherapeutic approaches and techniques integrated with practices such as breathwork, transcendental

meditation, yoga, and other Eastern meditative practices in order to facilitate insight, management of stress and anxiety, coping, and wellness.
Many clinicians are moving toward including these techniques into
practice (see, for example, Chapter 6 by Craig Cashwell).

In this regard, it is also important to mention several newer approaches
within the traditional psychotherapies themselves that are taking a new
look at potential spiritual elements. Some of these include revised psychological approaches to treatment and recovery in the addictions. For
example, Alan Marlatt (1999, 2002), a well-known cognitive behavioral
psychologist, has been working recently to include Buddhist meditation
in his practice of recovery therapy and relapse prevention. Others working at the interface of spirituality and the addictions include Christina
Grof and her work exploring "spiritual emergencies" (Grof, 1993; Grof &
Grof, 1989), and investigations of "quantum change" within psychology
and psychotherapy by William R. Miller and others (Miller & C'de Baca,
2001). Interested readers should examine the recent special issue of *In
Session/Journal of Clinical Psychology,* with Miller serving as Guest Editor,
for a good introduction to quantum change and its connection to addiction studies and spiritual conversion (Volume 60, No. 5, May 2004).

• The cultural disenchantment with materialism and the promises of
  modern science, leading to "spiritual hunger in an age of plenty"
  (Myers, 2000).

Moore (1992), quoted at the beginning of this chapter, states it
starkly: "The great malady of the twentieth century, implicated in all of
our troubles and affecting us individually and socially, is 'loss of soul'"
(p. xi). This is part of a larger cultural critique that has arisen at the end
of the twentieth century and is intensifying in the early twenty-first. In
this critique, the promises of modern society *and* modern science have left
us wanting. While many benefits have come our way, we have also become spiritually rootless—in the words of one keen observer, "spiritually
homeless" (Steere, 1997). In an "age of plenty" we remain "hungry," and
perhaps more confused and restless than is healthy.

David Myers, in a cogently written and keenly argued treatise, *The
American Paradox: Spiritual Hunger in an Age of Plenty* (2000), makes the
case that not only in the United States but around the world, we are approaching a spiritual crisis. While in advanced societies we are blessed
with many achievements, material benefits, wealth and power, nevertheless we live with gnawing doubts about the quality of our common
life and the worth of our attempts at meaning-making. As Vaclav Havel

(1994) has said, "the relationship to the modern world that modern science fostered and shaped now appears to have exhausted its potential. . . . The relationship is missing something." In these early days of the twenty-first century, the rise of religious fanaticism may be one attempt to supply that missing something but at the same time provides growing confirmation of the risks of narrow religious fundamentalisms, a breakdown of civility, and increased violence in the name of religious authority (ó Murchú, 1998). The crisis, it seems, is all around us.

There is, in short, out of all this hunger and crisis a contemporary search for the spiritual!

• The ongoing effects of renewal within mainline Christianity as a catalyst for renewed dialogue with science and the modern world.

In the 1950s and 1960s a number of the mainline Christian denominations began a fundamental reorientation in their stance toward modernity. On January 25, 1959, when Pope John XXIII announced his intention to call an ecumenical council of the Catholic Church, few understood how deeply transformative such an event would be. Yet it deeply shaped the global community as well as the internal dynamics of the Catholic community and the interrelationships within mainline Christian traditions.

Itself a response to a number of initiatives that were already taking place within Christianity, and often led by Protestant scholars, such as the new biblical scholarship that was occurring through dialogue with disciplines such as hermeneutics and historical criticism, the Second Vatican Council fashioned a new relationship between the Christian churches and the modern world. It became a catalyst for ecumenical dialogue within Christianity and with other religious traditions, many of which had sent invited representatives to the sessions as observers and active participants in the conversation. It was the impetus needed for renewed dialogue between religion and science. It highlighted the need for renewed interest in spirituality among all women and men of good will. Vatican II, in its dialogue with the modern world, established relationships, ecumenical and interdisciplinary, that continue to bear fruit in mutual dialogue and attention. It is one of the cultural roots of the contemporary interest in spirituality.

As the dialogue (between religions and between religions with the modern sciences) has moved forward, concerns with diversity, faith and justice, and the importance of grounding a vision of persons and social action in spirituality became more and more present in the conversation. Care of whole persons, including traditions of soul care, worked its way back into the dialogue with, and consciousness of, the modern world.

• The need to work effectively within a multicultural context, sensitively attending to clients' diverse ethnic, cultural, and value backgrounds (Burke & Miranti, 1992; Frame, 2003; Fukuyama & Sevig, 1999).

The exponential increase in diversity of this country's population has stimulated the understanding that clients' backgrounds are shot through with values, religious themes, spiritual orientations and experiences, biases, and so forth. Clients expect that their values, as well as their ethnic and cultural experiences, including spiritual events and understandings, will be honored and even utilized in the therapeutic context. The importance of recognizing a broad cultural and societal movement here should not be missed. We are at a pivotal moment of change in our paradigms for counseling and psychotherapy, in which we can acknowledge and develop new ways of thinking about the significance of values (including spiritual values), the role of culture, and the importance of a more holistic conception of what it means to be fully human (Bergin, 1992). Spirituality in counseling, to some degree an outgrowth and extension of multicultural awareness, is a critical component of this new paradigm. It is a "fifth force" within the clinical disciplines.

Daya Singh Sandhu in Chapter 4 and elsewhere speaks eloquently of counseling's sensitivity to spirituality as a fifth force movement, deeply impacting a variety of clinical disciplines and approaches (Stanard, Sandhu & Painter, 2000). Earlier forces, such as awareness of psychodynamics (first force), the powerful perspective of behaviorism (second force), and the impact of humanistic concerns (third force), are well understood to have had far-reaching implications for the understanding of clinical work. More recently, multiculturalism, understood as the fourth force in counseling and psychotherapy, has captured the imagination and sensitivities of practitioners and scholars alike. While there is ongoing discussion about the interrelationship between multicultural and spiritual sensitivities (Pate & Bondi, 1992), it seems clear that the topic of counseling and spirituality can and should be studied in its own right.

Within clinical assessment, treatment planning, and intervention, many health-related approaches now incorporate attention to ethnicity and culture, as well as to the values and spirituality expressed in these dimensions of living. Clinical tools such as the cultural (Hardy & Laszoffy, 1995) and spiritual (Frame, 2000) genogram are now in use. A number of survey and interview assessment instruments are also being developed, and some rediscovered from the field of psychology and religion (Gorsuch & Miller, 1999; Hill & Hood, 1999; John E. Fetzer Institute, 1999). These approaches can be seen as complementary and distinguishable.

- The rise of attention to women's issues, especially with regard to post-trauma experience and survivorship, as well as recovery of a sense of women's leadership, and connected concerns with ecology and care for the earth (Conn, 1986; Estes, 1996; Hessel, 1996; Ruether, 1992).

Contemporary sensitivity to women's stories and attention to issues of trauma and recovery in women's lives has sensitized all of us to women's needs in our society. This sensitivity has also resulted in highlighting the paths women take to recovery, mentoring, and leadership. Many of these paths are spiritual ones and lead to exploration of spiritual lifestyles and practices—old and new. This doorway into spirituality has captured the imagination of many in our society; it has created fertile ground for a more general exploration of the spiritual as a response to modern maladies.

Herman (1992) speaks of those whose spiritual path takes them toward social action as a way to reclaim authority and a positive self-image in the face of trauma and victimization. Social action allows traumatized persons to become "survivors" and reacquire a "mystical" sense of connection to others (p. 208). We often now see women finding a similar kind of spiritual dimension in a turn toward wiccan, Celtic, Native American, or Eastern spiritualities, and offering their experience for others in published works, workshops, conferences, and varying kinds of spiritual direction (Estes, 1996). For some women (and for some survivor men!) this spiritual journey also results in reclaiming minority or subjugated spiritual traditions within their own religious heritage.

Many spiritual paths are also allied with spiritual and theological notions about ecology, the victimization of the earth, and the value of a renewed creation-centered spiritual practice (Hessel, 1996; Fox, 1991 & 1983). Here again, earth-oriented spiritualities (such as Native American traditions) have become a popular and influential movement within contemporary culture. They have helped to sensitize both counselors and potential clients to the importance of spirituality in living.

- Influence of group movements, including Twelve Step fellowships (Steere, 1997).

Robert Wuthnow, in a series of studies (1992, 1994), presents a compelling picture of the resurgence of interest in spirituality. Wuthnow believes this interest is channeled into individuals' involvement in caring behaviors and small-group networks. Forty-five percent of Americans regularly engage in voluntary service, providing care in churches, shelters, civic groups, and so forth. In addition, 40 percent of all Americans, he says, are involved in small groups that meet regularly and provide mutual caring and support (reported in Steere, 1997, pp. 27–28). Perhaps the best known of the small groups is the wide variety of Twelve Step fellowships across the country. These fellowships, the core of a large recovery movement that emphasizes spiritual growth and development, have not only promoted the integration of spiritual perspectives into clinical care, but they have also drawn the attention of practicing clinicians to the (potential) "active ingredients" or "agents of change" they employ. These Twelve Step fellowships are clear in stating that these agents are spiritual in nature and effect.

Although small-group dynamics and the support of caring others are important elements in recovery from addiction, it is also hard to avoid the clear testimony of recovering persons and respected scientists alike that a spiritual vision and lifestyle are at the core of recovery (Mercadante, 1996; Miller, 1999; Morgan & Jordan, 1999). The cultural phenomenon of the Twelve Step movement has become another motive for spiritual interest and expectation among counseling consumers.

- A "stance of practicality," given the contemporary search for and worldwide reorientation to considerations of the sacred (Morgan, 2000; Steere, 1997).

What do we know about the yearning of people for inclusion of spiritual perspectives in their care?

Many people who come for counseling today bring with them a spiritual or religious worldview of some kind; many find their involvement in religious groups or spiritual movements to be meaningful. They expect counselors and therapists to understand and include their worldviews in the clinical process. Also, as more and more people become disenchanted with modernity, they look at traditional "modern" counseling and psychotherapy with a jaundiced eye. They expect that today's caregivers will meet their needs, not just for physical or mental health and the absence of illness, but for spiritual development and holistic healing as well. The data is persuasive and has been consistently demonstrated in recent years:

- Eighty-eight percent of the world's population follows some kind of theistic belief system (Frame, 2003, p. xi).

- Ninety-six percent of Americans claim to believe in "God, or a universal spirit," while 84 percent believe in a personal God accessible through prayer (Myers, 2000, p. 260).

- From 1994 to late 1998, the number of Americans feeling a need to "experience spiritual growth" rose from 54 percent to 82 percent (Myers, 2000, p. 260).

- Seventy-six percent of those who attend church report thinking at least a "fair amount" about "your responsibility to the poor," as opposed to 37 percent of those who rarely attend.

- Eighty-one percent of respondents in the Gallup poll in 1992 preferred some integration of their beliefs and values into the counseling process.

- Two-thirds of those responding, when faced with a serious problem in living, would prefer to be counseled by someone who personally holds spiritual values and beliefs (Kelly, 1995, 34).

- Fifty percent of elderly Gallup poll respondents wanted their doctors to pray with them as they faced death, and 75 percent said that physicians and therapists should address spiritual issues as part of their care.

Given this information, it is important for clinical professionals to examine their own perspectives, as well as the needs and expectations of clients. Professionals must then respond accordingly.

Those who come for counseling today clearly want us to respond to them with clinical competence and spiritual sensitivity. Yet, as described in the Preface, all of us in the mental health disciplines are just now learning how to do this. We are finally paying attention! The integration of spirituality into counseling and psychotherapy has been called for in recent years, but only now is really being addressed.

This book is an attempt to assist those who are interested in examining the integration of spiritual issues in clinical practice. It presents the experience of eleven professional counselors as they attempt to integrate spiritual concerns, issues, and values into their clinical work. The book provides a number of personal narratives from these counselors and psychotherapists discussing how they came to understand the importance of the issue and how they began to incorporate these concerns into their practice. Each contributor tells a personal story of a spiritual search, and of the journey to integrate spirituality into professional counseling practice. Chapters present casework from each contributor, suggesting ways to begin the process.

## References

ASERVIC. (1997). *Spirituality: A White paper of the Association for spiritual, ethical and religious values in counseling.* Available at *www.aservic.org/.*

Beers, C. W. (1944). *A mind that found itself.* Garden City, NY: Doubleday.

Benner, D. G. (1988). *Psychotherapy and the spiritual quest.* Grand Rapids, MI: Baker Book House.

Bergin, A. E. (1992). Three contributions of a spiritual perspective to counseling, psychotherapy, and behavior change. In M. T. Burke & J. G. Miranti, (Eds.), *Ethical and spiritual values in counseling* (p. 515). Alexandria, VA: Association for Religious and Value Issues in Counseling (ARVIC).

Boisen, A. (1960). *Out of the depths.* New York: Harper & Row.

Boisen, A. (1936). *The exploration of the inner world: A study of mental disorder and religious experience.* New York: University of Pennsylvania Press.

Browning, D. S. (1987). *Religious thought and the modern psychologies: A critical conversation in the theology of culture.* Philadelphia: Fortress.

Burke, M. T., & Miranti, J. G. (Eds.). (1992). *Ethical and spiritual values in counseling.* Alexandria, VA: Association for Religious and Value Issues in Counseling (ARVIC).

Cabot, R. (1908). The American type of psychotherapy. In W. B. Parker (Ed.), *Psychotherapy: A course of readings in sound psychology, sound medicine, and sound religion.* New York: Center Publishing Co.

Cabot, R., & Dicks, R. (1936). *The art of ministering to the sick.* New York: Macmillan.

Carr, A. (1988). *Transforming grace: Christian tradition and women's experience.* New York: Continuum.

Chandler, C. K., Holden, J. M., & Kolander, C. A. (1992). Counseling for spiritual wellness: Theory and practice. *Journal of Counseling and Development, 71,* 168–175.

Conn, J. W. (Ed.). (1986). *Women's spirituality: Resources for Christian development.* New York: Paulist.

Cornett, C. (1998). *The soul of psychotherapy: Recapturing the spiritual dimension in the therapeutic encounter.* New York: Free Press.

Ellison, C. W. (1983). Spiritual well being: Conceptualization and measurement. *Journal of Psychology and Theology, 11,* 330–340.

Engel, G. L. (1980). The clinical application of the biopsychosocial model. *American Journal of Psychiatry, 137,* 535–544.

Estes, C. P. (1996). *Women who run with the wolves.* New York: Ballantine.

Fox, M. (1991). *Creation spirituality: Liberating gifts for the peoples of the earth.* San Francisco: HarperSanFrancisco.

Fox, M. (1983). *Original blessing: A primer in creation spirituality presented in four paths, twenty-six themes, and two questions.* Santa Fe: Bear & Co.

Frame, M. W. (2003). *Integrating religion and spirituality into counseling: A comprehensive approach.* Pacific Grove, CA: Brooks/Cole.

Frame, M. W. (2000). The spiritual genogram in family therapy. *Journal of Marital and Family Therapy, 26,* 211–216.

Frank, J. D. (1963). *Persuasion and healing: A comparative study of psychotherapy.* New York: Schocken Books.

Fukuyama, M. A., & Sevig, T. D. (1999). *Integrating spirituality into multicultural counseling.* Thousand Oaks, CA: Sage.

Garrett, M. T. (1996). Reflection by the riverside: The traditional education of Native American children. *Journal of Humanistic Education and Development, 35,* 12–28.

Gorsuch, R. L., & Miller, W. R. (1999). Assessing spirituality. In W. R. Miller (Ed.), *Integrating spirituality into treatment: Resources for practitioners* (pp. 47–64). Washington, DC: American Psychological Association.

Grof, C. (1993). *The thirst for wholeness: Attachment, addiction, and the spiritual path.* San Francisco: HarperCollins.

Grof, S., & Grof, C. (1989). *Spiritual emergency: When personal transformation becomes a crisis.* Los Angeles: J. P. Tarcher.

Hardy, K. V., & Laszoffy, T. A. (1995). The cultural genogram: Key to training culturally competent family therapists. *Journal of Marital and Family Therapy, 21,* 227–237.

Hart, T. (2002). *Hidden spring: The spiritual dimension of therapy* (2nd ed.). Minneapolis: Fortress.

Havel, V. (1994, August 1). "Post-modernism—The search for universal laws." *Vital Speeches of the Day,* p. 613.

Herman, J. L. (1992). *Trauma and recovery: The aftermath of violence—from domestic abuse to political terror.* New York: Basic.

Hessel, D. T. (Ed.). (1996). *Theology for earth community: A field guide.* Maryknoll, NY: Orbis.

Hill, P. C., & Hood, R. W., Jr. (Eds.). (1999). *Measures of religiosity.* Birmingham, AL: Religious Education Press.

Holifield, E. B. (1983). *A history of pastoral care in America: From salvation to self-realization.* Nashville: Abingdon.

Ingersoll, R. E. (1995). Spirituality, religion, and counseling: Dimensions and relationships. *Counseling and Values, 38,* 98–111. Reprinted in M. T. Burke and J. G. Miranti, *Counseling: The spiritual dimension* (pp. 5–18). Alexandria, VA: American Counseling Association.

James, W. (1902). *Varieties of religious experience.* New York: Random House.

John E. Fetzer Institute (1999, October). *Multidimensional measurement of religiousness/spirituality for use in health research: A report of the Fetzer Institute/National Institute on Aging Working Group with additional psychometric data.* Kalamazoo, MI: Author.

Kelly, E.W. (1995). *Spirituality and religion in counseling and psychotherapy: Diversity in theory and practice.* Alexandria, VA: American Counseling Association.

Kleinman, A. (1989). *The illness narratives: Suffering, healing, and the human condition.* New York: Basic.

Kleinman, A. (1988). *Rethinking psychiatry: From cultural category to personal experience.* New York: Free Press.

Kleinman, A. (1980). *Patients and healers in the context of culture: An exploration of the borderland between anthropology, medicine, and psychiatry.* Berkeley: University of California Press.

Kurtz, E. (1999). The historical context. In W. R. Miller (Ed.), *Integrating spirituality into treatment: Resources for practitioners* (pp. 19–46). Washington, DC: American Psychological Association.

Lake, M. G. (1991). *Native healer: Initiation into an ancient art.* Wheaton, IL: Quest Books.

Larson, D. B., Swyers, J.P., & McCullough, M. E. (1997, October 1). *Scientific research on spirituality and health: A consensus report.* Bethesda, MD: National Institute for Healthcare Research.

Marlatt, G. A. (2002). Buddhist philosophy and the treatment of addictive behavior. *Cognitive and Behavioral Practice, 9,* 42–50.

Marlatt, G. A., & Kristellar, J. L. (1999). Mindfulness and meditation. In W. R. Miller (Ed.), *Integrating spirituality into treatment: Resources for practitioners* (pp. 67–84). Washington, DC: American Psychological Association.

May, R. (1939). *The art of counseling: How to gain and give mental health.* Nashville: Cokesbury.

McNeill, J. T. (1951). *A history of the cure of souls.* New York: Harper.

Mercadante, L.A. (1996). *Victims & sinners: Spiritual roots of addiction and recovery.* Louisville, KY: Westminster John Knox.

Miller, W. R. (1998). Researching the spiritual dimensions of alcohol and other drug problems. *Addiction, 93,* 979–990.

Miller, W. R. (Ed.). (1999). *Integrating spirituality into treatment: Resources for practitioners.* Washington, DC: American Psychological Association.

Miller, W. R., & C'de Baca, J. (2001). *Quantum change: When epiphanies and sudden insights transform ordinary lives.* New York: Guilford.

Miller, W. R., & Delaney, H. D. (Eds.). (2005). *Judeo-Christian perspectives on psychology: Human nature, motivation, and change.* Washington, DC: American Psychological Association.

Moberg, D. O. (1986). Spirituality and science: The progress, problems, and promise of scientific research on spiritual well-being. *Journal of the American Scientific Affiliation, 38,* 186–194.

Moberg, D. O. (1984). Subjective measures of spiritual well-being. *Review of Religious Research, 25,* 351359.

Moberg, D. O. (1971). *Spiritual well-being: Background and issues.* Washington, DC: White House Conference on Aging.

Moberg, D. O. (1967). The encounter of scientific and religious values pertinent to man's spiritual nature. *Sociological Analysis, 28,* 22–33.

Moberg, D. O., & Brusek, P. M. (1978). Spiritual well-being: A neglected subject in quality of life research. *Social Indicators Research, 5,* 303–323.

Moore, T. (1992). *Care of the soul.* New York: HarperCollins.

Morgan, O. J. (2002). Spirituality, alcohol and other drug problems: Where have we been? Where are we going? *Alcoholism Treatment Quarterly, 20,* 61–82.

Morgan, O. J. (2000). Counseling and spirituality. In H. Hackney (Ed.), *Practice issues for the beginning counselor* (pp. 170–182). Needham Heights, MA: Allyn & Bacon.

Morgan, O. J. (1999). "Chemical comforting" and the theology of John C. Ford, S.J.: Classic answers to a contemporary problem. *Journal of Ministry in Addiction & Recovery, 6,* 29–66.

Morgan, O. J., & Jordan, M. (Eds.). (1999). *Addiction and spirituality: A multidisciplinary approach.* St. Louis: Chalice Press.

Myers, D. G. (2000). *The American paradox: Spiritual hunger in an age of plenty.* New Haven: Yale University Press.

Oden, T. C. (1984). *Care of souls in the classic tradition.* Philadelphia: Fortress.

Ó Murchú, D. (1998). *Reclaiming spirituality: A new spiritual framework for today's world.* New York: Crossroad.

Paloutzian, R. F., & Ellison, C. W. (1984). Loneliness, spiritual well-being, and quality of life. In L. A. Peplauand & D. Perlman (Eds.), *Loneliness: A sourcebook of current theory, research, and therapy* (pp. 224–237). New York: Wiley-Interscience.

Pate, R. H., & Bondi, A. M. (1992). Religious beliefs and practice: An integral aspect of multicultural awareness. *Counselor Education and Supervision, 32,* 108–115. Reprinted in M. T. Burke & J. G. Miranti (1995), *Counseling: The spiritual dimension* (pp. 169–176). Alexandria, VA: American Counseling Association.

Peck, M. S. (2003). *The road less traveled, 25th anniversary edition : A new psychology of love, traditional values and spiritual growth.* New York: Touchstone.

Peck, M. S. (1998a). *Further along the road less traveled: The unending journey toward spiritual growth.* New York: Touchstone.

Peck, M. S. (1998b). *The road less traveled and beyond : Spiritual growth in an age of anxiety.* New York: Touchstone.

Peck, M. S. (1978). *The road less traveled: A new psychology of love, traditional values and spiritual growth.* New York: Simon & Schuster.

Rieff, P. (1966). *The triumph of the therapeutic: Uses of faith after Freud.* New York: Harper & Row.

Ruether, R. R. (1992). *Gaia and God: An ecofeminist theology of earth healing.* San Francisco: HarperCollins.

Schneiders, S. M. (1990). Spirituality in the academy. In B. C. Hanson (Ed.), *Modern Christian spirituality: Methodological and historical essays* (pp. 15–37). Atlanta, GA: Scholars Press.

Stanard, R. P., Sandhu, D. S., & Painter, L. C. (2000). Assessment of spirituality in counseling. *Journal of Counseling & Development, 78,* 204–210.

Steere, D. A. (1997). *Spiritual presence in psychotherapy: A guide for caregivers.* New York: Brunner/Mazel.

Stinnett, N., & DeFrain, J. (1985). *Secrets of strong families.* Boston: Little, Brown & Co.

Torrey, E. F. (1986). *Witchdoctors and psychiatrists: The common roots of psychotherapy and its future.* New York: Harper & Row.

Wilbur, M. P. (1999a). The rivers of a wounded heart. *Journal of Counseling & Development, 77,* 47–50.

Wilbur, M. P. (1999b). Finding balance in the winds. *Journal for Specialists in Group Work, 24,* 342–353.

Witmer, J. M., & Sweeney, T. J. (1992). A holistic model for wellness and prevention over the life span. *Journal of Counseling & Development, 71,* 140–148.

Wulff, D. M. (1997). *Psychology of religion: Classic and contemporary.* New York: Wiley.

Wulff, D. M. (1996). The psychology of religion: An overview. In E. P. Shafranske (Ed.), *Religion and the clinical practice of psychology.* Washington, DC: American Psychological Association.

Wuthnow, R. (1994). *Sharing the journey: Support groups and America's new quest for community.* New York: Free Press.

Wuthnow, R. (1992). *Rediscovering the sacred.* Grand Rapids, MI: Eerdmans.

❧

# CHAPTER 2

# "They Come to Us Vulnerable": Elements of the Sacred in Spiritually Sensitive Counseling

## Oliver J. Morgan

The voice at the other end of the phone sounded slightly annoyed and guarded. It was at the same time schmoozy, gruff and . . . world-weary. I wondered if the speaker really had, in the words of Alcoholics Anonymous, become "sick and tired of being sick and tired."

"Hello, Doc. This is Richard Gladstone. I believe Dr. Collins told you I would call."

"Yes, Mr. Gladstone. I expected to hear from you. What can I do for you today?"

"Gerry [Dr. Collins] feels it would be good for me to see you for a few sessions."

"As I remember, Gerry told me that you have been having trouble with relapse, that you'd been attending AA but felt you needed something more. He said that you thought some work on spirituality might be helpful. Do I have that right?"

"Yes. He said you would be someone I should talk to about that."

"Okay. I understand that you will still be seeing Gerry for on-going counseling and that he's recommending a consultation with me. Let's set up a time to see how we might work together."[1]

---

[1]The case vignette that follows is a combination of work with several clients over the years. It is a reconstructed conversation with details chosen to exemplify themes I believe to be important in

Richard was a forty-five-year-old man when he came to see me several years ago. He was a man of some accomplishments, successful as a financial advisor and involved in his community. His relationship with his wife and family was still intact, but they clearly wanted him to get help for his drinking problem.

It didn't take long into the first session to realize the other challenging elements in his "problem-saturated story." Richard had turned to alcohol use early in life, medicating the pain of growing up in a family with an alcoholic father and a chronically depressed mother. He was the middle child of five, and his achievements in high school, college, and business were routinely overlooked. He overlooked them, too. Richard spared no opportunity to tell me about his low self-esteem, bouts of depression, issues with authority and anger, and loss of "honor" through the deceptions he practiced in the face of frequent relapse. His guilt, shame, and anger at himself over the most recent relapse were palpable.

Richard was confused about his recurrent relapses. Although he had had some difficulty with alcohol in college, he had changed course and remained essentially sober through his early professional and marital life, having only an occasional beer or glass of wine. Over the previous seven or eight years, his drinking had escalated until he realized that he needed to stop. This time, however, stopping proved to be more difficult. He had begun attending AA, but was unable to maintain more than five or six months (and sometimes less!) of sobriety at one time. Then he would relapse. He had yet to put together a year clean and sober.

Richard and I worked together on a consultation basis for fourteen months while he continued in therapy. His therapist worked on individual, marital, and medication issues. I was free to work with him on relapse and issues of spirituality. Our initial sessions utilized both motivational interviewing (Miller & Rollnick, 2002) and transtheoretical or "stages of change" (Prochaska, Norcross & DiClemente, 1994) approaches.[2] We enumerated his reasons for quitting and potential benefits. We explored the resources he could martial to aid in this goal and the challenges to living out what

---

a consideration of counseling and spirituality. The vignette does not cover many of the more clinical interventions used in these cases, but focuses on spiritual elements. Disguises are used to protect the identity of the clients involved, who have read this vignette and consented to its use.

[2] For a clearly stated integration of these two contemporary approaches, see DiClemente & Velasquez (2002).

he wanted to accomplish. I listened carefully, affirming his earlier successes and reflecting back his expressions of desire for change. We identified some mechanisms and patterns that led to relapse in the past and constructed some strategies that he could put into place for relapse prevention. We worked on his sense of confidence in the face of this important life task.

Our early work utilized elements of willingness or readiness to change, mindfulness about the goals for change and the "causes and conditions" that underlie one's problems, and hope or confidence about the task—all essential conditions for change to occur and remain. I see these as "natural healing factors" in recovery (Edwards, 1984; Vaillant & Milofsky, 1982) and deeply spiritual in their essence, although they don't often sound precisely "spiritual" to clients. Willingness, mindfulness, and hope are core spiritual elements in a process of healing that requires collaboration and work. They form the ground or platform for the work of recovery (May, 1988 & 1991; Miller & Rollnick, 2002).

As this early phase drew to a close, Richard was about three months sober and entering a time of year that had been risky for relapse in the past. Now, however, when asked about his hope or confidence for reaching a year or more of sobriety, he could say "about a seven or eight on a scale of ten." This was improvement. Richard wanted more, and asked for more explicit work on spirituality.

I asked Richard to relax and visualize someone who he thought was the most spiritual person he had ever known. "My grandfather," he said. I then walked Richard through a simple guided imagery and visualization exercise in which he met his grandfather, who was deceased, and talked with him about his life and the challenges currently facing him. He experienced again his grandfather's presence, the smell of his aftershave, and the love in his eyes. Richard reconnected with many of his grandfather's best qualities. When the exercise was completed, we processed it together.

"Richard, what was it about your grandfather that led you to think of him as 'the most spiritual person' you've known? What qualities did he possess that let you know he was 'spiritual'?"

"I don't know really. He had a great sense of humor, even in the face of difficult circumstances. He created this sense of safety around him, like a warm blanket; I remember feeling protected when he would visit. He was calm, mellow; not in some wimpy or weak way . . . I saw him angry sometimes, especially about my father . . . but he would come to a place where he trusted that things would be okay. And, that's what he lived out of. He didn't live out of anger, but out of calm . . . and hope!"

"And those are qualities you think of as 'spiritual'—humor in the face of difficulty, safety, calmness, hope?"

"Yes, those and honor, you know, dignity in the face of living."

"Are those spiritual qualities you would like to have?

"Oh, yeah."

"See, Richard, I think that talking about spirituality in general is a good thing, but I am much more interested in what each person sees as the spiritual quality or challenge that faces him or her right now . . . this person, particularly, in the day to day. So, if you were to pick one of those 'spiritual' characteristics, what one do you feel you most need in your life now?"

"Honor. We've talked about this before, I know. But, I'd really like to live without deceit, without a double life. I'd like to live with dignity."

"Okay. Good. Now, what do we need to do for you to feel like you're getting there? And, what are you willing to do?"

Much more happened in our work together. At my suggestion Richard conducted an overall review of his life, as suggested in AA's Twelve Steps and as a way to establish a baseline for a new life of dignity. He discussed the results of this inventory with his AA sponsor and with me. He came to a place of greater acceptance about his life. He also came to a deeper appreciation of the psychological and emotional roots of his difficulties. He came to terms with old demons of fear in the face of helplessness as his family of origin was coming apart, and needs to assert control in the face of hopelessness, even if it was a self-defeating form of control (drinking). As our consultation work came to a close, he was over a year clean and sober, and ready for a new life in sobriety.

At our last session there was a sense of exhilaration and confidence.

"I feel good about what's happened, Doc. Feel better about myself . . . confident that things will be okay. Not in a cocky sense, just confident."

"Richard, I felt when you first came in that you were ready to make the changes that needed to happen. And, as we worked together I, too, became more confident about your success. You know, often between sessions and sometimes before them, I take time to sit down and think about the people I'm seeing. I make a mental picture of them, call them to mind, and try to open myself to their story as I'm coming to understand it. Sometimes, I get a sense of what's needed next. Sometimes, I remember something I should inquire about or have forgotten. Often, I feel called simply to pray for that person."

"Really?" He was intrigued.

"As we've worked together, you and I, I've often prayed for you between sessions and I've pretty much always felt you would succeed."

He looked directly at me—not a frequent occurrence—and smiled.

"I have come to believe that there is another presence in the room with us when I work with people, something or someone that wants the best for them.[3] I believe that God works in our lives, sometimes in unseen ways to bring the best out of even difficult or painful situations. I believe that's happened with you. My job is to assist and get out of the way."

"I'm really grateful for what we've done, for what's happened. I'll keep trying."

"I know you will."

## Who Am I?

This case presents what, for me, have become a number of salient themes in my current understanding of spirituality and counseling. Before I discuss some of these elements, however, I want to acquaint the reader with important aspects of my own life and social location. How did I get to be where I am?

I have been a marriage and family therapist, professional counselor, and counselor educator for over twenty years. I am currently chair of the CACREP and CORE accredited counseling programs at my university. I am a life-long Roman Catholic and a former member of a religious order, the Society of Jesus (or Jesuits), for over thirty years. I was also a leader in my church as an ordained priest. As such, I learned and lived a distinct tradition of spirituality (Ignatian), practicing a brand of active contemplation and discernment, which has nourished me all my life. This spiritual formation was the catalyst and crucible in which my desire to work clinically took shape; I became a clinician and counselor as my way to do ministry.

---

[3]Goethe said something similar: "There is one elementary truth, the ignorance of which kills countless ideas and splendid plans: that the moment one definitely commits oneself, then Providence moves too. All sorts of things occur to help one that would never otherwise have occurred." Quoted in Miller & Rollnick (2002, p. 3).

In my work as a priest, I came to value the role of counseling skills and approaches to pastoral care. I wanted to know more and to practice competently. I wanted to incorporate clinical ways of thinking and working into my ministry. While my intention was to learn to work clinically, the motivation for doing so was almost entirely religious and spiritual. It was natural then to seek training that could integrate the two. I found a comfortable fit within pastoral counseling and psychotherapy.

Interestingly, the field of pastoral counseling was undergoing its own change of identity at that time, moving from a more clinical orientation to a focused integration of spiritual and religious identity (Jordan, 1986). Boston University, where I chose to study and train, was a focal point of this new perspective. Those years of pastoral-clinical formation were important, as I learned ways to integrate the clinical and pastoral languages and commitments I had into a personal and professional style of practice. It was a very rich "interdisciplinary conversation" (Schlauch, 1995). However, the truth is that I have been drawn all my life toward relating spirituality and religion to human problems and the deep experiences of human living. The integration of spirituality and counseling has been a life task. Doctoral work deepened and refined this integration. Today, I continue to try to think and work in an interdisciplinary way, living "on the bridge" as a citizen of both the clinical and religious/spiritual worlds (Morgan & Jordan, 1999; Schlauch, 1995). This is a fruitful and life-giving way for me.

More recently, my life has taken some surprising turns. I loved the priestly work and am grateful for the opportunities for study and professional development. I loved the Jesuits and still do. Nevertheless, at the age of forty-nine, I felt called to "leave" their company and begin a new phase of life as a husband and father. In this process, I am learning a great deal more about counseling, and spirituality, and love. Now, as a layperson in the church, and someone with many clinical and professional credentials as well as a spiritual background, I am still captivated with the task of integrating these themes from my life. What follows is something of a statement—still a work in progress—about what I have learned so far.

## A Sense of Posture and Place

As a seasoned practitioner, I try to come to each new counseling relationship with an awareness of who I am, and what the client(s) and I are about. I believe that what we actually do and the skills we bring to the task are, as in so many other areas of life, a function of what we *think* we are doing. Clinical action follows from clinical identity. My current professional identity and conceptualization of the work are the products of my life-long and ongoing pastoral and clinical conversation, and are at the heart of my professional commitments.

I regard the work of counseling as a sacred privilege, and I see both the place where I work and the counseling relationship itself as a sacred space. It is within this context that clients and I have the opportunity to engage in authentic relationships and to encounter their ground in a mysterious I-Thou core that graces and works with us. It is ultimately this double-edged encounter, and the perspectives and skills that facilitate it, that heal. Perhaps a biblical story can suggest the power of this, as I understand it. Such stories illuminate dimensions of our work that might remain otherwise hidden.

The story of God's initial encounter with Moses at the burning bush comes to mind (Exodus 3:1–4. 17).[4] Moses, a person with his own challenging history and vulnerabilities, along with a disability of speech, sights a rare phenomenon and moves to investigate. After telling Moses from the "burning bush" to "put off your shoes for this is holy ground" (*haqqodesh* in Hebrew), God refuses to hear that Moses' "disability" will impede him in the task that God is going to give him. He will become God's spokesperson on behalf of the people! Toward the end of the story, God does agree to an "accommodation," providing Moses' brother, Aaron, as a helper in public speaking, but the task that will give Moses' life new meaning and purpose remains.

What intrigues me about this story, aside from the Cecil B. DeMille quality of the encounter, is that at the end we are left to wonder whether the "ground" referred to is "holy" because God alone is there, or whether the place is "sacred" because it is the place of encounter between God and a vulnerable, wounded human being. Over time I have come to a sense of what I believe to be true.

I believe that the counseling or consulting room is a sacred space. It is the place of encounter, where clients come to us with their pain and vulnerabilities. We try to attend to the client "at the place where his or her soul is on the line" (O'Reilley, 1998). The clients who come to us—individuals, couples, families, groups—come to us "vulnerable." It is our privilege to work collaboratively with them in order to increase health and healing. This is a sacred task. When viewed in this way, the counseling room can be the place in which life stories are told, authentic encounter

---

[4] I am grateful to Rabbi Michael Levy (1995) and to Gerald May (1991) for elements of interpretation around this classic Exodus story.

is sought and encouraged, and change—perhaps even transformation—is facilitated (Barrett, 1995). This is a way of seeing the counseling relationship as a "healing alliance" and "holding environment" with a distinctly spiritual twist (Morgan, 1987).

I believe that the Hebrew and Christian scriptures are full of stories that address the issue of holiness precisely in God's desire to encounter human beings in need. Our counseling offices and the relationships we forge there are potential places of such encounter. As Hart says, "God is present and active in the therapeutic project, whether we advert to it or not" (2002, p. 7). Since this is so for me, I believe it is essential to place myself in a stance of openness and receptivity, not only to the client's life story but also to the presence and grace of God.

This core belief leads me to spiritual practices I have found deeply meaningful over the years. *Before* and *during* sessions, I try to remind myself prayerfully of these faith-oriented convictions, becoming mindful of the deeper clinical and theological dimensions of our situation (Morgan, 1987 & 2000; Morgan & Jordan, 1999). I try to work from a sense of God's care and hope for this person and our process of healing. In this way, I pray with, or in the presence of, my clients (see Frame, 2003).[5] In prayer, I believe that we come to a deeper awareness that our lives and the lives of our clients are embedded within a spiritual context of God's caring presence. This awareness deepens a sense of what we are about; it can also liberate us to experience new dimensions and resources for healing. Clients and I meet within the healing context of the "reign of God" (Morgan, 1987). The "reign [or kingdom] of God" is the biblical metaphor and foundation for a vision of the way human life and creation ought to be. It is a symbol of hope and a call to action on behalf of vulnerable persons. A vision of healing in view of God's kingdom can help to sustain spiritually sensitive counselors when the work becomes challenging.

I pray in another way as well. *Between* sessions, I routinely take time to clear my mind of distractions, calling each of my clients to mind and contemplatively trying to gather some sense of what they need. I also ask for the grace to be helpful. I have come to believe in this form of praying for clients between clinical encounters as setting the stage for a more mindful sense of what I am about. It also gives me a new perspective. I

---

[5]This is different from explicitly "praying with" clients out loud in vocal prayer. Frame (2003) suggests that this practice is both controversial and fraught with ethical concerns, although there may be situations in which it is appropriate. Her discussion of this (pp. 184-187) bears consideration by any thoughtful practitioner. I'm speaking here, however, about something quite different.

have found it to be liberating, in that I am reminded that I share responsibility for what happens. I am no longer "the healer" who carries the full, grandiose burden of the work; I am a collaborator, working together with clients and with God in the process of healing (Morgan, 1987).

In these ways my own life of prayer is enriched by integrating it with my professional identity and practice. Praying with and for clients becomes a kind of mindfulness meditation on professional and spiritual identity, as well as a way to open myself up imaginatively to the world of those with whom I work. It extends, refines, and grounds my caring.

At some point in our work together, it is not uncommon for me to tell clients that I pray for them like this. This is one way in which I invite discussion of spirituality. Telling clients that I pray with and for them can be viewed as a kind of self-disclosure that is nonthreatening. They can dismiss it or regard it as quaint, if they choose. It is, however, a simple statement about one way in which I regard our work together. Most often, I find that clients are touched, or curious, or relieved. If clients react positively to such an invitation, I then inquire directly about how they view their difficulties from a more explicitly spiritual point of view. Does prayer make sense to you in this situation? How? Do you think of God as with you in all this? How might God be with and for you in this struggle? What might be the most loving or life-giving thing to do here?[6]

These inquiries are different from, and deeper than, specific questions about one's religious tradition of origin and the supports or challenges one receives from a community of faith (such as Were you raised Catholic? What church, if any, do you currently attend? Do you find your current religion helpful for living?). Questions about religion of origin, clients' experiences with religion, and the benefits or struggles one receives from religious traditions are important opening questions in any clinical encounter, I believe. Marsha Wiggins Frame (2003) devotes an entire chapter in her text, *Integrating Religion and Spirituality into Counseling,* to the issue of assessment. She thoroughly discusses the importance of assessing these spiritual and religious issues through intake forms, clinical interviews, spiritual genograms, instruments exploring spiritual experiences and beliefs, and other formats (see also Morgan, 2002; Sperry, 2001; Stanard, Sandhu & Painter, 2000). I believe it is important to cover these issues in a routine, matter-of-fact way early in the

---

[6]For a full presentation of such a perspective in pastoral counseling from a Roman Catholic point of view, see Hart (2002). Since in the case study Richard was interested all along in developing spirituality and came to me for that purpose, it was unnecessary to use this approach earlier in counseling.

clinical process. They can be easily covered in initial assessment forms or intake conversations.

However, as one delves more deeply in the counseling relationship, I believe it may also become appropriate to explore the role of spiritual beliefs (such as providential care or views of an afterlife), spiritual practices (such as prayer), and ways of making meaning spiritually (as in God's presence or the role of love) that may be important to the client. Throughout the process of counseling, practitioners ought to be sensitive to potentially spiritual issues and should inquire about them. Understanding clients' spiritual and religious experiences and perspectives is every bit as important as understanding the sexual, familial, and developmental elements of their lives. Taking the initiative to ask about these topics opens up the possibility for clients to discuss them as part of counseling.

As a believer in the essential role of spirituality for healing and health, I attend to spiritual ways of doing this work in conjunction with sound clinical theory and practice. The fundamental viewpoint I bring to counseling and spirituality suggests that, as whole human beings with cognitive, affective, behavioral, conative, and spiritual dimensions, we deserve a healing process that honors the whole of us (Benner, 1988). I have also come to believe something that Robert Wubbolding proposes, namely that we are all "spiritual beings with specifically local experiences" (2000, p. 27). Concreteness is important.

With Richard, I used an approach that refocuses the clinical discussion of spirituality from generalities to concrete, specific (local), and "actionable" particulars. The imaging exercise and follow-up recounted above is a tool I've learned from work with individuals and groups struggling with addiction, and have refined in presentations to a variety of health care practitioners.[7] The exercise has several parts to it. Following a guided visualization framed around the concept of "a spiritual person I've known," the counselor engages individuals or groups in conversation about spiritual qualities that were noticed, what the individual(s) find attractive or compelling about these qualities, what the individual(s) believe is needed here and now, and in planning some strategy around developing these qualities. This exercise creates a broad space within which conversation can occur, experiences and values can be discussed, and action plans can be developed. The exercise can set an agenda for change that client and counselor will monitor. It is a particularly

---

[7] I am grateful to Lew Abrams, former Clinical Director at Marworth, a drug and alcohol rehabilitation center in Waverly, PA and to Ellen Morgan, counselor at the University Counseling Center in Scranton, PA for their inspiration and help in developing this approach.

helpful way to expand upon early clinical discussions that revolve around stages and motivation for change, while staying focused on a spirituality that is grounded and concrete.

I have used this approach with different clients and groups over several years. The approach has evolved over time. Clients find it a relatively easy and nonthreatening way to identify and work with spirituality. I am often amazed at the variety of "spiritual qualities" that emerge from clients' experiences and the depth of the stories that accompany these qualities. Just about everyone, even those alienated from traditional religion, finds this an easy way to connect with spiritual themes.

## Spiritual Platform

I have come to believe that as caregivers, we must assess the spiritual environment we (co-) create in our work. All too often, we are unaware or uncritically accepting of this element of our work. Yet, an environment *is* created. Harry Aponte (1999), a remarkable family therapist, speaks directly to this point:

> Attending to the spiritual aspects of clients' personal struggles calls for awareness by clinicians of the spiritual environment they create in their therapy. All therapy rests on a spiritual platform of values and philosophical outlook that reflects the spirituality of the clinician, that is, his or her moral standards, sociopolitical convictions, and religious outlook. . . . The spiritual platform they construct will support or undermine, contribute to or detract from the spirituality of their clients. The therapy will help shape people's solutions to their problems and thereby the spiritual quality of their lives.  (1999, p. 81)

Aponte elaborates on this "spiritual platform" in ways that any counselor can resonate with. He speaks of beliefs the counselor brings to practice, such as beliefs about people's ability to change; the potential of adversity to promote change;[8] the healing and restorative power of relationships, however damaged and complicated; the intrinsic health of reliance on others and God, or a higher power. He speaks of values and orientations the counselor brings, such as what we judge to be

---

[8] I'm reminded of Carolyn Vash's classic 1994 work, *Personality and adversity: Psychospiritual aspects of rehabilitation.*

healthy or sick, fruitful or unfruitful goals for counseling, worthy or un-worthy ways of living, the value of confronting past pain or working with broken relationships. He speaks of the foundations upon which we base an ethical approach to our work (such as "at least, do no harm;" "do unto others . . ."). All these elements, deeply spiritual in nature, guide clinical action.

Do counselors believe that people can turn their lives around in the face of, or perhaps because of, hardship? Do they believe that people can change themselves even if they cannot change their circumstances, and that it is worthwhile doing so? Do they believe that people can do the right thing no matter what the cost? Do they have faith in the power of love to restore even deeply flawed relationships? Do they encourage taking stands for love, forgiveness, connection, justice, community, or hope? The realities these questions point to form a spiritual fabric or platform for our work in counseling.

Aponte also reminds us that a critical element in the spiritual platform is the spirituality of the client (1999, pp. 79–82). What are the clients' answers to the questions above and will the morality, worldview, religious beliefs, deepest desires, hopes, and loves of the client be respected?

Once clients know and experience that their spirituality—their story of graces, and wounds, and sins; of gifts and growing edges; of hopes and desires—can be an active part of their therapy and a platform for our work together, they are then fully free to express their souls, that is, who they really are and aspire to be. When spirituality is part of best practices in our work, both the spirituality of the counselor and of the client come to the encounter and the spiritual platform of care is co-constructed. This makes for a lively, nourishing, and even sacred encounter.

## Spirituality as Forging a Spiritual Life

In the contemporary search for clear definitions and operational concepts about spirituality, it is easy to forget that what we are talking about here is the living of a spiritual life. This is not the same thing as religious commitment to a set of beliefs and rituals, to an historical church com-munity, or to a denominational structure and its leaders. Spirituality is about living spiritually. This requires a certain amount of mindfulness about who we are and what we are about. It also requires collaboration with grace, that enabling and transforming power to live life fully (May, 1988 & 1991).

I have come to believe that grace or graciousness is always coming to us. God constantly addresses and invites us into health and into relationship.

We "swim in an ocean of grace" (Morgan & Jordan, 1999, p. 252). However, it is easy to forget this most essential fact about ourselves, and it is difficult to collaborate consistently with the grace that comes our way. Collaboration with grace, and the love it breeds, is what I mean by living a spiritual life. This takes us into the realm of spiritual practices and disciplines. Richard and I had a head start in this area because of his interest in recovery spirituality. The Twelfth Step of AA makes it clear that there is a discipline and a lifestyle involved in recovery spirituality:

> Having had a spiritual awakening as the result of these steps, we tried to carry this message to alcoholics and to practice these principles in all our affairs.   (Alcoholics Anonymous World Services, 1957)

A spiritual awakening is expected to appear as the result of following a disciplined and principled Twelve Step path. Most awakenings do not come easily. They require work as well as grace and can fade if not nurtured. Incorporation of spiritual (such as prayer, self-examination, meditation) and other healthy practices (such as exercise, service, a balanced schedule of work and play) into a revised lifestyle is essential for therapeutic change. In working with recovering people, I have learned the value of incorporating life disciplines and practices into all the counseling I do. This highlights the role of client action and collaboration in his or her own project of healing.

Richard came to our consultation already persuaded about the need for change and about the value of the Twelve Step approach. In this approach, an entire spiritual discipline, a recovery project, is laid out. One engages in this project by joining and participating in a group, working with a sponsor, and engaging in the discipline of the Twelve Steps. This discipline moves the individual through a succession of traditional spiritual practices (that also happen to make good clinical sense; see DiClemente, 1993; Twerski, 2000), including developing a sense of willingness and readiness to change (Steps 1–3), engaging in extensive self-examination and confession to others (Steps 4 and 5), humbly accepting oneself (Steps 6 and 7), taking direct action to alter one's lifestyle and rectify past mistakes (Steps 8 and 9), committing oneself to ongoing personal development and change (Steps 10 through 12) as well as service to others (Step 12). This is a pretty muscular form of spiritual development. It demands a full change in lifestyle over the long term in order to change one's behavior (such as drinking or drug use). It recognizes that both addiction and recovery are lifestyles with bio-psycho-social *and* spiritual dimensions. Perhaps the most strenuous aspect of this recovery work is the need for self-examination and confession. This personal review, or what is called a "moral inventory," has long been part of many forms of spirituality. The goal is not to induce guilt or engage in moralistic self-flagellation. Rather, the purpose is to arrive at a balanced assessment of one's life and to stir both motivation for and guidance in self-change. It is a deeply spiritual exercise. I believe that it should be conducted prayerfully, from the perspective of God's (higher power) view of the person.

With Richard, I encouraged him to fulfill this Twelve Step suggestion by working to catalogue his strengths and personal weaknesses or "growing edges" as he believed God saw them. Journaling and writing out lists of strengths and "edges" became his disciplines for this project. I also encouraged him to prayerfully ask for help in this task. He began hesitantly at first, but soon warmed to the project. Richard found that as he sat down and cleared his mind for this work, thoughts and ideas would come to him. He found himself feeling grateful for these insights. This allowed him to reclaim a sense of reliance on his Higher Power, as they worked together prayerfully—from his point of view—to develop a balanced view of Richard's life, while setting an agenda for continued growth in the spiritual life. After all, the strengths and challenges he was reviewing, along with his view of the "causes and conditions" of his addiction and relapse, would be his unique set of challenges for the rest of his life.

Understanding his personal set of challenges and strengths set an agenda for Richard as a collaborator in his own growth. In my experience, the issues that underlie one's addiction continue to confront the person long into recovery. They set the terms for engagement with life and for ongoing spiritual and personal development. It is important to note that Twelve Step approaches envision a penetrating search for the underlying roots of the conditions that drive addiction. AA literature speaks of "self-will run riot" and "self-centered fear" as two of the likely suspects, the mainsprings of addiction. Richard needs to understand the mechanisms that drive *his* addiction. He also needs to get a handle on the triggers and the cognitive-behavioral cycle that lead to relapse for him. Becoming more mindful—as I've said, another spiritual concept!—of the factors and vulnerabilities that drive this person's addiction and contribute to relapse risk is part of the work of successful recovery (Dodes, 2002).

Richard had identified one particular emotional response that seemed to be toxic for him and led to risk for relapse. This was his anger when confronting situations in which he felt he was being controlled or taken advantage of interpersonally. As we explored this, he wondered aloud about "some prayer or practice that could help me through the anger . . . a way to deal with it." Knowing he was in recovery, I asked if he ever used the "serenity prayer." He said that he did, but that his grandfather had referred to a form of the prayer that was longer and richer. He expressed a wish to know more about that.

I gave him a copy of the longer form, attributed to the Reverend Reinhold Niebuhr and adopted by AA (Alcoholics Anonymous World Services, 1957):

> God grant me the serenity to accept the things I cannot change, the courage to change the things I can, and the wisdom to know the difference. Living one day at a time; enjoying one moment at a time. Accepting hardship as the pathway to peace. Taking as my Lord did this sinful world as it is, not as I would have it. Trusting that He will make things right, if I surrender to His will. That I may be reasonably happy in this life, and supremely happy with Him forever in the next.

He was delighted and told me afterwards that he had given a copy to his mother, who confirmed that his grandfather had relied on it.

Over a period of several months, Richard worked to make time for this prayer in his daily routine. At first, he set aside time in the middle of the day to sit back, collect his thoughts in the midst of busy activities, and quietly say the prayer, mulling over its meaning. (This form of classic meditation worked for him.) As the weeks went by, he found himself remembering to recite the prayer when he was anxious, or angry, or even in moments of joy. He found this simple spiritual practice gave him balance. He found it became a quiet companion during his day. More importantly, he discovered that it framed a growing relationship.

Before turning to the deeply relational aspect of spirituality, however, I want to remind the reader that the living of a spiritual life is a cognitive, affective, behavioral, and conative enterprise. That is, spirituality affects our thinking and feeling, our actions and choices. It is not so much another dimension of life alongside others; it grounds and suffuses all the others. It appeals to every part of us as human beings. Twelve Step spirituality, indeed all forms of spirituality, envision a transformation of the person and the life that he or she lives. This is why the entrance into recovery is described, as it is in so many other spiritual traditions, as an "awakening" or is seen as the result of a "conversion" (Morgan, 1992;

Morgan & Jordan, 1999). Those in recovery are called to new ways of thinking, acting, and living. Indeed these individuals are invited into a new lifestyle. A transformation of vision and lifestyle is what the Twelve Steps promote (Morgan, 1992), and I have come to believe that such transformation is the result of opening oneself to spiritual practices and a spiritual way of life.

Nothing is ever really the same again.

## Spirituality as Relationship and Connectedness

In speaking of spiritual awakening and living, the question is logically asked: Awakening to what? To whom? This is the last element of spirituality I want to address.

A paraphrase that has been attributed to the pastor Jonathan Edwards holds meaning for me in this regard: Spirituality is "a posture of one's very being that allows seeing not different things, but everything differently" (Ernest Kurtz, 1999, Personal Communication). People who try to live spiritually and with awakened hearts do not see a world that is different from the one the rest of us see. They see the world with different eyes, like those who are in love. They see through the world to the love that holds it together. This new way of seeing is essentially a contemplative gaze or approach to life and work that incorporates the awareness of God's presence and activity in all of life (May, 1991).

> Let us love the actual world that never wishes to be annulled, but
> love it in all its terror, but dare to embrace it with our spirit's
> arms—and our hands encounter the hands that hold it.[9]

What I and others have experienced is that such a contemplative approach to life leads one to a surprising revelation, namely that God, or one's higher Power, or whatever one sees as ultimate in life, is *not* passive. Rather, each of us is sought and invited, not just to deeper insights, or a new perspective, or into religious practices, but into relationship! I have come to believe that spirituality is about a living, growing relationship with one's higher power. This relationship conditions and opens out into all others, forging a web of connectedness that leads the individual to care for, love, and serve others. Relationship is the motivation that drives

---

[9]Quote attributed to Martin Buber in Gerald May's chapter on "Contemplative Presence" (1991, p. 191).

a revision of lifestyle. A loving relationship with God is the core and driving force of a spiritual life.

As a lifelong Catholic Christian and follower of Ignatian spirituality, I think of spirituality as developing and living a relationship of love with a personal God. The entire thrust of Christian spirituality is to develop such a relationship, just as Jesus himself spoke of his Father in intimate, personal terms. St. Ignatius, the founder of the Jesuits and their spirituality, also spoke of developing such a relationship, speaking of prayer as "one friend speaking with another." *The Spiritual Exercises* of St. Ignatius, a fundamental text for followers of Ignatian spiritual traditions, has as its goal the "finding of God in all things" (Ganss, 1991). The Christian mystical and monastic traditions, as is true of many other religious traditions, speak likewise of a personal relationship with God. Beyond rituals, dogmas, beliefs, and practices, the core of many religious traditions, as the vessels or milieu for spirituality, is a relationship with the Divine. This is the living, breathing heart of spirituality.

It is hardly surprising, then, that my take on spirituality and counseling begins from this point of view. While I understand that some religious traditions do not have this personal element, it is a very alive notion in my life. Spirituality for me involves a personal experience of and relationship with God, that leads to ongoing development of a spiritual way of living, and a set of viewpoints or beliefs about the ways in which spiritual concerns weave themselves into living and professional practice (such as sacred space, sacred task, spiritual environment, and outlook). Spiritual practices open one up to, and nourish, this way of living.

In a study of long-term recovering alcoholics (Morgan, 1992), I discovered that for many of them the founding moment of recovery was understood as a moment of intervention and grace, pulling them out of the vicious cycle of addiction. Those who experienced this "saving moment" also spoke about a deep and abiding experience of being personally cared for, of feeling themselves as benefactors of providence. Over time in recovery, they described a deepening sense of trust, acceptance, and providence—not simply confined to the past but extending into their current everyday life. They described a sense of guidance and protection in living, a sense of simple and familiar relationship with the Higher Power of their recovery. Many called it God; others did not. But the sense of trust and hope, of "miracles happening," and quiet confidence that they and their loved ones would be cared for, were unmistakable. They experienced themselves as "listened to," and God or Higher Power as "approachable." They staked their recoveries and their lives on this relationship.

Richard began to experience many of these same feelings as he found ways to deepen his life of prayer. Over time he became more comfortable with himself, more at peace and less dominated by his anger. He attributed this to his growing relationship with God, rooted in his recovery program and his use of the Serenity Prayer. He spoke of himself as "just another bozo on the bus," human and accepted.

It is important to note that relationships such as this give rise to a radically different sense of self and world, and become the catalyst for desires to return the gift received in recovery. It becomes the ground for altered experiences of others and for service to them. The relationship becomes a fundamental source for changes in lifestyle.

## Concluding Thoughts

I have spoken in this chapter about ways I understand the connection between spirituality and counseling. I have tried to lay out a view of spirituality that is both accurate to my life story and personally meaningful to me. I have also tried to provide examples of how spirituality can be viewed in the practice of professional counseling.

Perhaps it is only fair to acknowledge that what I believe and have written here challenges me to keep developing myself both professionally and spiritually. For me, this means continually developing myself clinically and staying in touch with the religious and spiritual roots of my own commitment to professional counseling as a healing art. It also means continuing to develop a life of prayer, of relationship with God and others. It means exploring traditional and new spiritual practices and disciplines that keep my spirituality alive. Finally, it means honoring the spirituality that my clients and I bring to the task we have together.

For readers of this chapter, let me suggest that, while I believe openness to spirituality in counseling is rewarding, I also believe it demands hard work. Those interested in pursuing this integration in their own practice must become familiar with the growing literature that is out there, beginning with the list of "spiritual competencies" published by the Association for Spiritual, Ethical, and Religious Values in Counseling (ASERVIC). This list emerged from a "Summit on Spirituality," sponsored by ASERVIC, a division of the American Counseling Association (ACA). A copy of the competencies is included in the appendix at the end of this book.

Interested readers must also engage in their own personal exploration of spiritual roots, history, and beliefs—culminating in a commitment to ongoing spiritual development and practice. They must, in addition, find their own way to incorporate this approach into professional practice and monitor their progress with high-quality supervision, at least in the beginning. As professionals, integrating spirituality into our practice makes a claim on us to continue our own personal and professional development. Spirituality, I believe, allows us to "see everything differently." At least on my best days, as I look at the world, I see everything as tinged with the holy. From the needs of my next client to the joy in my daughter's eyes, everything is sacred. We are all blessed by God, who searches for us and loves us from the heart of the world.

This is both a gift and a responsibility. And I am grateful for it!

## References

Alcoholics Anonymous World Services. (1957, 1985). *Alcoholics Anonymous comes of age: A brief history of A.A.* New York: Author.

Aponte, H. J. (1999). The stresses of poverty and the comfort of spirituality. In F. Walsh (Ed.), *Spiritual resources in family therapy* (pp. 76–89). New York: Guilford.

Barrett, R. L. (1995). The spiritual journey: Explorations and implications for counselors. In M. T. Burke & J. G. Miranti (Eds.), *Counseling: The spiritual dimension* (pp. 103–111). Alexandria, VA: ASERVIC/ACA. [Originally published in *Journal of Humanistic Education and Development, 26,* 154–163.]

Benner, D. G. (1988). *Psychotherapy and the spiritual quest.* Grand Rapids, MI: Baker Book House.

DiClemente, C. C. (1993). Alcoholics Anonymous and the structure of change. In B. S. McCrady & W. R. Miller (Eds.), *Research on Alcoholics Anonymous: Opportunities and alternatives* (pp. 79–97). New Brunswick, NJ: Rutgers Center of Alcohol Studies.

DiClemente, C. C., & Velasquez, M. M. (2002). Motivational interviewing and the stages of change. In W. R. Miller & S. Rollnick (Eds.), *Motivational interviewing: Preparing people for change* (2nd ed., pp. 201–216). New York: Guilford.

Dodes, L. (2002). *The heart of addiction.* New York: HarperCollins.

Edwards, G. (1984). Drinking in longitudinal perspective: Career and natural history. *British Journal of Addiction, 79,* 175–183.

Frame, M. W. (2003). *Integrating religion and spirituality into counseling: A comprehensive approach.* Pacific Grove, CA: Brooks/Cole/Thomson Learning.

Ganss, G. E. (Ed.). (1991). *Ignatius of Loyola: The spiritual exercises and selected works.* New York: Paulist.

Hart, T. (2002). *Hidden spring: The spiritual dimension of therapy* (2nd ed.). Minneapolis: Fortress.

Jordan, M. R. (1986). *Taking on the gods: The task of the pastoral counselor.* Nashville, TN: Abingdon.

Kelly, E. W., Jr. (1995). *Spirituality and religion in counseling and psychotherapy: Diversity in theory and practice.* Alexandria, VA: American Counseling Association.

Kurtz, E. (1999). Personal communication.

Lake, F. (1987). *Clinical theology: A theological and psychological basis to clinical pastoral care.* New York: Crossroads.

Levy, M. (1995). To stand on holy ground: A Jewish spiritual perspective on disability. *Rehabilitation Education, 9,* 163–170.

May, G. G. (1991). *The awakened heart: Living beyond addiction.* New York: HarperCollins.

May, G. G. (1988). *Addiction and grace: Love and spirituality in the healing of addictions.* New York: HarperCollins.

Miller, W. R., & Rollnick, S. (2002). *Motivational interviewing: Preparing people for change* (4th ed.). New York: Guilford.

Morgan, O. J. (2002). Alcohol problems, alcoholism and spirituality: An overview of measurement and scales. *Alcoholism Treatment Quarterly, 20,* 1–18.

Morgan, O. J. (2000). Chapter 11: Counseling and spirituality. In H. Hackney (Ed.), *Practice issues for the beginning counselor* (pp. 170–182). Boston: Allyn & Bacon.

Morgan, O. J. (1992). In a sober voice: A psychological study of long-term alcoholic recovery with attention to spiritual dimensions. *Dissertation Abstracts International, 52* (11), 6069B. [University Microfilms No. 92-10480.]

Morgan, O. J. (1987). Pastoral counseling and petitionary prayer. *Journal of Religion & Health, 26,* 149–152.

Morgan, O. J., & Jordan, M. (Eds.). (1999). *Addiction and spirituality: A multidisciplinary approach.* St. Louis: Chalice.

O'Reilley, M. R. (1998). *Radical presence: Teaching as contemplative practice.* New York: Boynton/Cook.

Prochaska, J. O., Norcross, J. C., & DiClemente, C. C. (1994). *Changing for good.* New York: Avon.

Schlauch, C. R. (1995). *Faithful companioning: How pastoral counseling heals.* Minneapolis: Fortress.

Sperry, L. (2001). *Spirituality in clinical practice: Incorporating the spiritual dimension in psychotherapy and counseling.* Philadelphia: Brunner-Routledge.

Stanard, R. P., Sandhu, D. S., & Painter, L. C. (2000, Spring). Assessment of spirituality in counseling. *Journal of Counseling and Development, 78,* 204–210.

Twerski, A. J. (2000). *The spiritual self: Reflections on recovery and God.* Center City, MN: Hazelden.

Vaillant, G. E., & Milofsky, E. S. (1982). Natural history of male alcoholism: IV. Paths to recovery. *Archives of General Psychiatry, 39,* 127–133.

Vash, C. L. (1994). *Personality and adversity: Psychospiritual aspects of rehabilitation.* New York: Springer.

Wubbolding, R. E. (2000). *Reality therapy for the 21st century.* Philadelphia: Brunner-Routledge.

❧

# CHAPTER THREE

# "Where Our Spirits Touch": The Process of Counseling and Spirituality

## Clifford ("Ford") Brooks

Spirituality is dynamic and ever-changing, not static or immobile. It is a process of awareness that unfolds throughout each day of our lives. Trying to define spirituality is like holding water in one hand; it is present yet difficult to describe. The challenge in writing this chapter is that we were asked to do just that, define and describe spirituality and its application to clinical work. Each author was asked to address three questions concerning spirituality: What is our own definition of spirituality? How did we come to consider spirituality as significant in our clinical work? And finally, how did spirituality factor into clinical work with one of our clients?

I've written this chapter to address all three queries, and I've added a segment entitled "Core Clinical Concepts" of spirituality. The first section of this chapter addresses significant events in my life that have impacted my spiritual exploration. The core clinical concepts of spirituality highlight five areas I feel are important within the counseling realm. The middle section describes how I've found spirituality to be clinically significant, and I've highlighted areas of particular focus such as spiritual awakenings, spiritual sickness, and relapse. The final pages of the chapter describe Spencer, a client of mine who exemplified how our therapeutic work together addressed spirituality in counseling.

## What Is Spirituality?

I've come to believe that in order to address this topic, I first need to review my own life story and events, which have contributed to my personal understanding of spirituality. The conclusion of this review is a description rather than a definition. Although counseling literature provides multiple definitions of spirituality, I believe the idea defies definition. Spirituality is in the experiences and events of life, profound and mundane, which help us to understand our essence and soul. Ultimately, it is an individual and personal interpretation. That being said, I don't believe it is possible to truly address spirituality with clients without first exploring our own journey within this realm. As with multicultural counseling, examining ourselves first prior to addressing client spirituality is essential. Because of this belief, I've outlined life events from my childhood to present, which have contributed to my understanding of spirituality. Contributing to my own understanding are the many clients who, through their struggles with addiction and recovery, have taught me about life and spirituality. The combination of my own life experience and the stories shared by my clients continues to help me negotiate spirituality, in personal as well as professional practice.

### The Accident

The runway of my life began a year prior to my birth in 1961. On a lazy weekend afternoon in Chester County, Pennsylvania, my mother made a significant chance decision, which ultimately saved her life. In a flash, an immense Philadelphia Electric truck hit the right side of the convertible she was riding in, ripped off the roof of the car, and instantly killed my mother's friend in the passenger seat as well as one of the truck drivers. My mother's decision to sit behind the driver saved her life. The driver of the automobile lost her sight in one eye. My mother sustained two broken arms, one broken leg, and lost all of her front teeth. Just over a year later I was born, against all odds and predictions of her doctors. At a very early age I understood how my life was special.

### Religious Underpinnings

My earliest recollection of the word *spirituality* came through attending Sunday school at the local Episcopal Church. In college at the University of Richmond, I attended chapel services each Sunday, listening intently to Dr. Burhans as he delivered meaningful, nondenominational messages in which religion and spirituality were intertwined.

My first year in college was to bring a great deal of pain and joy. Within months of arriving in Richmond, my parents separated, my mother was diagnosed with breast cancer for the second time, and my father's alcoholism was in the later stages and completely out of control. During my first year, I pledged Sigma Chi Fraternity, an organization based on spiritual principles. The combination of chapel attendance and the affiliation with a group of men helped me connect with a higher power, which subsequently supported me through the rough curves of academic and personal struggles. In addition to chapel and the fraternity as places of spiritual solace, nature significantly added to my connection with a higher power. With that in mind, during my junior year I became a registered Maine fishing guide and worked for two summers at a fishing camp in Maine.

### "It's Not About Fishing"

In the middle of my first summer, I guided a father and son for one week. The father was in his early seventies and the son in his mid-forties. It was a week in which no matter what I did, we didn't catch fish. I enjoyed these two fellows, particularly the father who chewed tobacco and dribbled spit down his chin all day long. About halfway through the week, and after having boated no more than ten sizable fish, the son came over to me at lunch and said, "Ford, we've had a wonderful time here this week, and what makes it such a special time is that it will be my father's last. You see, he has leukemia and has little time left to live. This is our last father and son vacation." After hearing his words I recommitted my efforts to find as many fish as I could in the remaining days of their vacation, to make it their best vacation ever.

I tried every trick in the book, and visited every spot that I knew in the past had produced fish, but nothing seemed to work. The harder I tried, the less likely we were to get even a bite. I admitted my defeat and apologized for the poor fishing. On the last day, however, the father came up to me, with spittle all over his chin and shirt, and he said, "Ford, this has been a wonderful trip. I know you have worked hard looking for fish all week; however, catching fish is the least of what I was interested in. I've been out here in this great state of Maine with my son and you this week, and it has been wonderful. It's not about catching fish."

I was shocked. Not about the fishing? It then dawned on me how I missed the process that had been unfolding in front of me all week. I had been so busy trying to catch fish that I missed the point. It was clear how this gentleman knew the sunset of his life was near, where relationships with others and nature were paramount; fishing was not. I had witnessed a special and sacred moment between father and son in the wilderness.

Ironically, in 1989 I, too, experienced a most profound and moving point in my life. For as long as I can remember nature has been significant in my development; spiritually, emotionally, and physically.

## The Fish and the Owl

After two years of intensive care, steroids, colostomy bags, and numerous operations, my own father's spirit was well nigh gone. He had lost almost 100 pounds and looked gaunt. His eyes had sunk deep into his skull, and he was voicing his loss of will to stay alive. By now, he had stopped drinking; however, his other addiction would continue until his last breath. For over fifty years, he smoked three packs of unfiltered cigarettes per day. In fact, he ultimately needed only one match per day because he lit each cigarette with the one before it. His heart finally gave out. Although I knew it was inevitable, and certainly he lived much longer than any of us had expected, he was gone. His worn-out body was at rest and his spirit was at peace.

His final wishes were to have my stepmother and me scatter his ashes in a lake in the Poconos. After the funeral, we drove with his ashes down to the lake and slowly distributed them into the water. At that point, I was trying to make sense of it all and looking for some sign from God, nature, or the cosmos that there was meaning. As we watched the waves of sediment curl under the water, a fish jumped not thirty yards from the dock, and at the very same moment an owl hooted in the distance. It was a surreal experience; a fish and an owl making known their presence at the same time of my father's burial. They brought to me an understanding that my dad would be okay. Somehow, I felt that we were related by nature and connected with something greater. It was as if I were between the beginning and the end, the alpha (fish) and the omega (owl). I considered this to be a profound spiritual experience that has significantly influenced my life. Although I had continually found peace in nature, it was much clearer to me how nature played a major role in my connection with something greater and allowed healing to occur.

I came to understand that the fish represented life, and the owl represented death and wisdom. The synchronistic occurrences brought meaning to my father's death and to my life. Following this death experience, I began reading literature on Native American traditions. In my exploration, I came across an individual (Tom Brown) who wrote about his experience in nature and the profound impact on his life. His teachings and writings have been instrumental in not only processing my father's life and death, but also my own spiritual journey.

## The Tracker

Over the next five years, I attended three workshops by Tom Brown, known internationally as a tracker, teacher, and writer. He was mentored from age eight until his mid-teens by "Grandfather," an Apache Indian. Tom created a school to share with others what he learned from Grandfather and to help participants live with the earth, more simply, spiritually, and peacefully.

For three years, I ventured into the Pine Barrens of New Jersey for multiple weeklong workshops on Grandfather's philosophy as told by Tom. During those times, I experienced a connection with the sacred circle of life, which I humbly attempt to incorporate in my daily living and clinical work.

## Reflection

My mother's accident, my college experience, nature, and my father's death have been significant experiences, which have helped me develop spiritually in life. Whether those difficult times were a result of my choices or a matter of life circumstances, it almost always seemed darkest before the dawn of new light. In those times, I found myself physically on my knees, surrendering to a greater power, which I choose to call God. In retrospect, it was during those times when I felt most human, vulnerable, and humble. Those times have helped me appreciate the present moments and the simple pleasures of life.

Today is good. I am a father. The birth of Sarah, our child, is the beginning of a new life. Each day, I am in awe at the creation and cycle of life, where the spirit has ignited another soul in the world. And, in the same life, I've watched family and friends pass on. Their lives have taught me to appreciate my own life and to live each day to the full. I am keenly aware how that spirit of life can be gone in an instant. I am grateful for ALL that I have experienced and will experience, the good and the bad, the joy and the pain.

## Core Clinical Concepts

The following pages include ideas and concepts gleaned from the preceding stories, which I feel are pertinent to exploring spirituality with clients: Process versus Content, the Tao and the Paradox of Control, the Darkness Before the Dawn, and Surrender and Meaning in the Moment.

## Process versus Content

Yalom (1995) describes "process" in terms of the underlying story, the one behind the literal content or facts being presented. In Western culture, we tend not to live or converse on a process level, due to its awkwardness. Instead, we safely stay in the content of what is being expressed. Tapping into the process means we are willing and able to point out the possible deeper meanings and are willing to voice them. I believe cultivating this awareness helps clinicians in moving to the core of what may be unfolding in therapy with their clients.

A personal illustration of process versus content occurred over a period of time beginning in graduate school. Although much of my life I have been an observer, it wasn't until my Master's program that I voiced the hidden story behind the story that clients presented in the counseling office. This understanding of process was not sequestered to the counseling office; I also discovered it in nature.

One afternoon during a weekend hike, I decided to sit and relax by a spot on a hillside in the woods. The area was warm and comfortable, surrounded by a circle of light provided by a gap from the trees above. After thirty minutes or so of sitting and enjoying the sunshine, I realized my joy was brought about by the loss of trees in the forest around me. Only through the gap from the dead trees could the sunlight shine through. In order for life-giving light to penetrate, other trees had to die. For me, this was an experience of understanding the process in nature, seeing beyond the sunshine, to how it came about and a broader concept of what it meant.

The content in this example was sitting in the warming light. The process was what occurred in order for this to happen. It is through this process lens that, I believe, we are tapping into an energy or spiritual flow beyond the protective content. The spirit or life energy that runs through all things can also be described by the next concept: the Tao.

## The Tao and the Paradox of Control

The Tao is the ever-present flow of life energy that is everywhere. Many clients (and human beings in general) tend to fight against the Tao or "path." The times when we believe we are in total control are the times when our egos have taken over, and we are potentially headed for crisis.

The Tao cannot be controlled. It is considered spiritual, but not religious. It is the void and the nonvoid. When we surrender to the Tao, we have discontinued fighting the way or path. We are accepting on some level our powerlessness and lack of control. With surrender, we can simultaneously begin to gain control of our lives by letting go of what we cannot control and focusing on what we can begin to change (Wildish, 2000).

Control is an illusion, and, in fact, we have very little control over anything other than how we act on our feelings. It is typically when we are feeling most out of control that we attempt to show or indicate to the rest of the world that we are in control. The wisdom of the first three steps in Alcoholics Anonymous (AA) suggests surrendering to and acknowledging powerlessness and unmanageability, coming to believe that something greater can help bring about sanity, surrender, and letting go of control. It is at these times that we can be truly free. Many of our problems stem from our difficulty in knowing what we can and cannot control and from our resistance to surrender. For many of us it is most bleak prior to letting go. However, at the time of surrender comes freedom.

### Darkness Before the Dawn

I have found in my own life, as well as in the lives of my clients, that it tends to be very dark before the dawn of new light. I don't mean to imply that being in the dark is not painful and depressing. On the contrary, it is quite difficult to see the sunlight through the trees when one is immersed in this dark place. Trusting that life will be any better requires quite a leap of faith. For some, pain is an insurmountable obstacle. In the struggle through our deepest pain and vulnerability we come to understand fully our humanity, the frail state in which we live.

For a number of years, I worked with a treatment organization that had, as its representative coat of arms, a cluster of oak leaves in a circle. One of the leaves was green, followed by an even greener version. A colorful leaf was next, followed by a dark brown one. The circle ended and began again with the green leaf. This cluster of leaves represented where many clients begin their journey of healing and how they moved from death to life.

Sitting with clients during their moments of darkness is when the spirits of counselors can therapeutically touch those of their clients. Observing clients as they move from despair, isolation, and hopelessness into hopefulness, connectedness, and joy is powerful; this shift occurs at the time of surrender.

### Surrender and Meaning in the Moment

Addicted clients, early on in the recovery process, have begun the process of surrender and experience the feelings and thoughts of life moment-to-moment. Almost as if a bandage is quickly pulled from a wound, there now are vulnerabilities. Spirituality is not found somewhere else, although individuals may find solace and great peace of mind and heart in certain geographical places. Spirituality is within and around us each moment of the day. For recovering addicts/alcoholics, each day without a drink or a drug is a miracle. From gratitude comes a rare understanding of life, through addiction.

The first time I heard an individual say, "I'm Joe and I'm a grateful recovering alcoholic," I thought to myself, *You have got to be kidding. You're grateful for what? For all the pain and suffering your addiction has caused you and others?* Years later, I understood the wisdom of his words.

There is a parallel process in coming to understand this wisdom. In order for me to understand what this gentleman was saying, I had to come to terms with my own demons in life. I had to understand that in order to appreciate who I am today, the relationships in my life, and my spiritual program, I had to travel my own journey first. If I changed one aspect of my life, one choice or situation, I would not be who I am today. In effect, I believe this person was saying (paraphrased), "I'm Joe. For many years of my life I drank and drugged, not only destroying my relationships with others, but with myself. I've lost jobs, relationships, and money, but most of all self-respect. Now, in sobriety, I can face my behaviors, learn that I am not alone, trust in a power greater than myself, and outline my shortcomings and make amends to those I have hurt. Finally and continually, I will help others who are in pain from their addiction. If I change any of my history, I would not be the person I am today and I like that person. I can be free from the chains of addiction and be present for the miracles that occur each and every day in the relationships I have with friends and family."

## Spirituality as Clinically Important

When I started in my master's program in 1983, *spirituality* was an intriguing term to me, although I had done some personal exploration before that point. In the mid-1970s, the director of the program, Dr. Marcia Lawton, was forging a new frontier in the training of addiction counselors at Virginia Commonwealth University. It was also around the same time that certification for addiction counselors developed, and as a result, training programs were geared toward the Certified Addiction Counselors (CAC) credential.

A significant educational film, *Chalk Talk,* presented by Father Joseph Martin, an icon in the addiction field, and used in the master's program, helped bridge the gap between the spiritual program of Twelve Step recovery and treatment. Dr. Lawton's understanding of addiction and training of counselors was instrumental in my current practice and teaching of addiction courses and my overall philosophy of counseling due to the experiential nature of the entire curriculum. There has been much progress since that time with regard to research and pharmacological interventions, as well as varied treatment protocols. Yet the significance of spirituality in the growth and recovery of addicts remains the same.

From the very first overview class, I learned to view addiction from a holistic perspective with spirituality at the center of the recovery wheel. All other aspects of human potential existed in relationship to it. In addition to the theoretical learning in the program, we examined in each class our own use of alcohol or drugs, the impact on us of use by family or friends, and the myths and misconceptions of addiction in general. A majority of the students were either in recovery, were about to get into recovery, or had lived or were living with active addiction. Rarely was there a counselor in training who didn't have some personal experience with addiction.

The courses were designed to explore the above areas, and to do so experientially. For example, the group class was four days in length, and we lived together for the entire time. The family therapy class was three days in length, and in it we lived with our surrogate families and explored family dynamics. The recovery class not only reviewed the Twelve Steps but also focused on how they could work in our own lives. Additionally, in each class we were required to attend Twelve Step meetings and record our experiences. The program was very experiential and instrumental in my spiritual growth as a person. I found Twelve Step meetings to be genuine, honest, and powerful discussions, which helped me understand the wisdom of the Twelve Steps and of Alcoholics Anonymous. Most important, though, was the fellowship, support, and simplicity that helped me grow as a person and ultimately as a professional counselor.

This experiential aspect of the program was very beneficial, given that I had little experience with clients or with a family member who ever really got into recovery. So from a personal and a professional standpoint, self-exploration and meetings were crucial. In the Big Book of Alcoholics Anonymous (1976), reference is made to alcoholism being a "soul sickness." In addition to the physical aspect of addiction, the soul or spirit of the individual is also taken captive, thus hindering personal growth and sobriety. It was during this graduate school program that the interface of counseling and spirituality became a reality. Spirituality was clinically important because clients voiced its importance in their recovery. In addition to spirituality the use of counselor clinical interventions, theory, group therapy, and psychiatric consultation, was factored into effective therapy and treatment.

## Relapsing Clients and Spirituality

As I entered the field of counseling, I worked with articulate, intelligent, and creative clients who appeared to understand their addiction on a cognitive level. That perhaps was not enough, because many of them returned to treatment after relapsing, if they were fortunate. Gorski (1989) believes individuals may have a difficult time with lifelong sobriety if their recovery is limited to cognitive awareness. He contends that those individuals who are making changes cognitively, emotionally, physically, and spiritually have a better chance at remaining abstinent. Addressing spirituality is therefore important in relapse prevention.

In early sobriety, the physical nature of addiction tends to be paramount. This includes challenges with cravings, withdrawal, urges, and compulsive/impulsive behavior (Gorski, 1989). However, along with any necessary medical intervention, support and fellowship with others in recovery is critical, as may be spirituality. In his letter to Bill Wilson, Carl Jung expressed a belief that individuals needed to have a spiritual-religious experience and place themselves in a religious-spiritual environment if they were to get sober (Jung, 1974).

Clients have disclosed to me the difficulty in remaining sober early in their recovery. They described a sense of misery in wavering between not wanting to use and cravings urging them to use. Some were able to remain abstinent, despite the physical cravings and urges. Among those who were able to remain abstinent, I observed a number of consistently shared characteristics. The first was a willingness to be involved in some form of treatment. By treatment I mean some type of structure that had an ongoing program for the first six months to a year of recovery (such as inpatient, outpatient, partial programs). The second was attendance in Alcoholics Anonymous or Narcotics Anonymous meetings on a regular, sometimes daily basis, keeping them plugged into human contact/fellowship that they could not otherwise find. A final aspect was their willingness to explore the idea or concept of spirituality in recovery and openness to that which they could not find alone. This usually included a surrendering of ego and making connection with others.

Those clients who did not involve themselves with ongoing treatment, did not attend meetings regularly, or maintained the belief that they could conquer their addiction on their own, found themselves in and out of detoxification and treatment settings. Early on, I discovered the power of addiction and the mortality rates associated with it.

My first experience with a client dying occurred while I was working as an intern in a local hospital detoxification setting. Many of the clients I worked with were late-stage addicts and alcoholics needing three to five days of medical attention before they were referred to treatment. One patient who drank daily (one fifth of whiskey or more per day) was in detoxification for four days and referred to an inpatient facility for treatment. Against the wishes and recommendations of both family and staff, this patient left detoxification stating he could get sober on his own, that he was in control, and that treatment was not needed. Within four months he was dead, cirrhosis of the liver at age thirty-eight.

The above patient exemplifies the power of denial, cravings, and his disconnection from others (mental, physical, and spiritual components of the disease respectively) in combination. Despite the medical team's recommendations, this man drank again and died. Not only was he physically addicted, he was spiritually sick.

### Addiction as a Spiritual Sickness

At the core of each human being is a desire and a need to be loved by others as well as an ability to love others. When this capacity to love and be loved gets cut off, people lose touch and connection with the world around them. Addiction does just that; it takes its victims and isolates them from those they love most. Not one client ever expressed to me that, at their first use, they intended to become addicted or to isolate themselves from family and friends.

Consider clients who start smoking pot at the age of ten and by thirteen are drinking every weekend. If we were to go inside of those individuals, to their core spirit, we would probably discover lonely, sad, angry, and misunderstood thirteen-year-olds. Whatever the chronological age, the ability to love others or oneself is interrupted. Instead, the use of chemicals becomes the "center," the god, the way of being accepted—a very powerful connection. Take this child and multiply by three and now you have a thirty-nine-year-old client coming in after three decades of using drugs and alcohol. A tremendously powerful relationship has developed with chemicals over that time. That relationship of mind, body, and spirit is still very intricately organized around the principle of getting high no matter what the cost, though they may want to stop. Imagine the seemingly insurmountable challenges for clients to stop using. Then imagine this thirty-nine-year-old client actually stopping. This individual is now confronted with an internal void and emptiness which he or she is unable to fill without returning to use. At this point, individuals face a moment of truth. How can they live with this feeling and not go back to using the drug that has medicated the emotional pain for so long? Clients who are able to surrender to a process/power outside of themselves can potentially experience a sense of peace, relief, and connection.

My clients have shared with me over the years that surrendering and letting go of perceived control brings a sense of peace. Their collective experiences contribute clinically to my work with all clients. The idea of spiritual awakening (described in the following paragraphs) translated for many to a belief that they would have a profound and moving experience. Very few realized it was more likely to be a process of surrenders, letting go, getting out of the way, and receiving support. Somehow in their minds it was going to be a BIG event, and if it wasn't then they were not "getting it."

Ironically, it's the small surrenders that really contribute to a sense of freedom and serenity. Many times I heard, "Ford, I really don't get this God stuff. I go to meetings but I feel as though I will never get it." Yet, over time, as they attend meetings, and place their bodies, minds, and hearts in a room of honest and recovering individuals, they report a shift, not only in their thinking, but in their way of listening to themselves.

If clients wanted to attend alternative support groups, I would support anything that would place them in an environment where others were trying to grow in addiction recovery. I found, however, that many clients were just as resistant to attending alternative support meetings as they were to AA or NA meetings. The problem seemed to be more about their difficulty in surrendering their own will than about the particular support group they attended. The clients who refused outside help and had all the answers were the ones I tended to see repeatedly, usually in crisis. Although they were admitting their addiction, they were not admitting powerlessness over the drug, nor were they acknowledging the devastation their chemicals had brought forth. They blamed their drinking/drugging on their job, spouse, relationship, or just bad luck. These clients had difficulty in learning from their decisions and from their addiction. In essence, their ability to admit powerlessness and to verbalize a sense of humility was lacking. As a result, life of continued insanity, misery, and ultimately death was in store unless they were able to get sober.

## Spiritual Awakenings

Bill Wilson, co-founder of Alcoholics Anonymous, had what would be described as a profound spiritual awakening. In his hospital bed after many detoxifications, Bill W. was told by his physician, Dr. Silkworth, that his body could not withstand another binge on alcohol and that his life expectancy was quite short if he did drink again. Following his brief meeting with Dr. Silkworth, Bill described a bright light which engulfed the silent hospital room. He described a warm breeze blowing as he visualized himself atop a mountain with bright lights above, connected with beams of light. Bill described this as a profound and spiritual experience, which brought with it a number of understandings. The first was Bill's new awareness that in order for him to remain sober, he needed to seek out other alcoholics, for he saw the connected lights as a network of alcoholics helping other alcoholics. The second outcome of this experience was his loss of craving for alcohol (Kurtz, 1979).

For many entering Alcoholics Anonymous and hearing of this transformation, anything short of miraculous wouldn't be considered a "spiritual experience." The challenge for me and many of my colleagues in working with addicted clients was to help them recognize the "miracles" that occurred in their lives each day. Clients did not usually come into my office at the very beginning of treatment having a clear understanding of spirituality. They just wanted to stop using and start living a clean and sober life. The problem was that it wasn't easy. The adage that the Twelve Steps are a simple program for complicated people is certainly true for many of the clients I worked with in therapy. If there was a way of making their recovering lives more complicated, they certainly would find it. Spirituality often meant simplifying.

### Attending Twelve Step Meetings

By attending many Twelve Step meetings, I've found spirituality to be a significant factor in the lives of those in the rooms, particularly those with long-term sobriety. What better way to understand spirituality in the lives of addicted clients than to attend Twelve Step meetings? Talking to recovering people, listening to stories of what it was like and how it is now has most certainly helped me in my approach with clients. Listening to descriptions of the process of surrender happening over and over again, descriptions and stories of the process of letting go and the freedom it brought, has certainly impacted my work. Being the adult child of an alcoholic brought its own demons and roadblocks that I had to address before I was ever really going to help others. In that way, I was like many counselors who work with addictions. Personal experience, whether it be through their own addiction to drugs or alcohol, or through being raised or living with an addict or alcoholic, is potentially very helpful in understanding the internal process of recovery.

I understood for myself how the "ism" in my own life needed attention and how helping others would be a parallel process. The "ism" refers to the behavior, thoughts, feelings, and compulsions that need attention in recovery. The Big Book refers to liquor being a symptom of the alcoholism where individuals need to get down to "causes and conditions."

Recovery and the Twelve Steps address the "ism" where stopping is not the biggest problem; it is in staying stopped that the difficulties come into play. If we do not address the "isms" in our lives, how could we ever expect to help those who suffer with their addiction? In summary, how did I get into considering spirituality as clinically important? It started with my own internal exploration, followed by the experience of my clients. As I am able to see the changes and growth in my life, I can empathize with clients during their own incredible journey.

## Spencer

The conclusion of this chapter focuses on my work with a client (Spencer), and how spirituality was integral in his therapy and process of growth. I describe the aspects outlined in the preceding pages and discuss the implications in his treatment.

Spencer was a fifty-two-year-old Caucasian male referred to me by an inpatient treatment program. He had been in treatment twice before and involved in Alcoholics Anonymous during his episodes of sobriety. He arrived at my office open and willing for outpatient counseling. Unfortunately, his job required that he be out of town with great frequency, as he was one of a few individuals in the company who could address technical problems. At the same time, his employers were also concerned about his drinking, giving him an ultimatum after the second inpatient admission. He was instructed by his superior that if he were found drinking on the job again, he would automatically lose his employment. It was clear to Spencer what was on the line this time around.

His treatment plan consisted of daily attendance at Alcoholics Anonymous meetings, even when he was out of town. He obtained AA meeting lists in each of the cities where his company sent him. He also agreed to call me once per week for a twenty-minute session on the phone to discuss any particular cravings, problems, or concerns. When he was in town, we would meet for individual sessions, and he would continue attending AA meetings. Throughout counseling, Spencer was willing to explore the spiritual aspects of his recovery program. He was raised in the Catholic tradition, and found his belief in God, along with the Twelve Step program, crucial in his sobriety. He understood, as we reviewed his relapse history, how attempting to take back control of things not really in his power, the lack of humility, and defensiveness, were signs he was disconnecting from God and his spiritual program.

After two months, Spencer began missing his weekly phone calls to me. It was also not too long after the last phone call he was discovered drinking on the job, at which point he was terminated from employment. I always wondered if his drinking wasn't intentional so that he could get fired and spend more time at home with his family, so I asked him one day about this. He related that he indeed felt isolated and apart from those he loved, and that historically his drinking made decisions for him. Though unemployed, he was now home and could really focus on his recovery.

In our work together, he talked about his relationship with God and how, even though he drank, he felt a connection, however minimal. It was important for me to create an environment where Spencer could talk about his faith and upbringing in the Catholic tradition and how religion and spirituality for him were different. In his therapy he expressed religion as a structure for the worship of God, and AA as a spiritual program, utilizing God to maintain his sobriety. He threw himself back into meetings and attended therapy group and individual counseling on a weekly basis. He and his wife met periodically for couples sessions to address communication and trust issues. Spencer was able to keep his focus on the here and now, practice breathing and meditation at home, where he prayed daily for strength to remain sober.

Much of the time, therapy focused on his feelings and experiences in the moment. My orientation in both group and individual counseling with Spencer accentuated his emotional, spiritual, and physical experiences during the therapy hours. His emotional communication with his wife and children grew, and eventually he found employment closer to home. Ironically, his job loss brought about new life, again reinforcing the death-loss life cycle. Through his pain came an understanding of his joys and an ability to give back to others struggling with their sobriety.

Through our work together, I felt Spencer became alive again. In group sessions he was reflective and able to identify and share his feelings with other men. He managed to put together a year of continuous sobriety, the first in his life. I felt very fortunate to have been there with him through the rough times. His recovery was truly a miracle.

After I had been in private practice for a number of years, an opportunity presented itself, and I was at a crossroads in my own life. I was offered a full-time teaching position in another state where I would become a counselor educator. The decision to leave my practice and become a professor was the most difficult professional decision I've ever made. It meant closing out with all of my clients, one of whom was Spencer.

Our final meetings were filled with reflection and sadness. Spencer said goodbye to me and his group, agreeing to maintain contact through AA, a promise he kept . . . until his death a year later. He had fought most of his adult life with alcoholism and finally achieved continuous sobriety and a joyful life, only to be diagnosed with cancer. Spencer finally "got it," and then moved on.

## Breathing

There are a number of approaches I took with Spencer during our work together, which I felt were important to his spiritual growth. One of these was helping him focus on breathing. We spent time in individual counseling and in group sessions, practicing slow breathing, focusing on each breath, and bringing his attention into the moment. As discussed earlier, the Tao exists everywhere and breathing helps to understand the ebb and flow of that energy. Essentially, we are not separate but connected. I would ask Spencer to close his eyes and visualize his breath as it moved down his throat and into his chest and out his mouth. At points, I would ask him to take a deep breath and exhale slowly, which helped him focus and allowed him to utilize this technique when he was distracted or upset outside of the therapy session.

I regularly played soft music when facilitating breathing exercises and on occasion I used silence in place of music. The musical selections I used with Spencer consisted of soft melodies devoid of lyrics. The music of New Age artists (flute, chimes, drums, guitar, and synthesizer) helped to create a meditative and relaxing environment for breathing, and subsequent guided imagery exercises.

## Guided Imagery

Another approach was to use guided imagery with Spencer. In conjunction with the breathing exercise, I used guided imageries to create a safe place for Spencer to relax and connect with his higher power/spirit. A favorite guided imagery I used with Spencer entailed the creation of a meditation circle in his mind's eye. This creation was important as he developed a method to relax and connect with his meditation spot. I would talk Spencer through the entire guided imagery and then discuss it at the end. In order to reach the meditation circle in his mind, I would instruct Spencer to close his eyes and visualize walking along a pathway until he came upon a set of stairs to the right. I asked him to walk down each step until he faced a large arch. At his pace he would walk through the arch and into his meditation circle. I asked him to visualize walking to the meditation area and sitting in the middle of the circle. I would ask him to visualize light, warmth, and peace descending upon him in the circle—all of this as he sat quietly in my office with his eyes closed. I would facilitate his return to the path and to the room where he would slowly open his eyes and discuss the experience with me. I encouraged Spencer to practice this visualization at home and gave him a transcript of the guided imagery.

## Spirituality Group

One of the groups that Spencer participated in was called the spirituality group where members talked openly about their struggles, questions, and reflections on God, higher power, nature, and so forth. This forum of open discussion helped Spencer negotiate his guilt feelings and shame from his addiction. In conjunction with group discussion, I used some of the methods described above (breathing, music, and guided imagery) and, periodically, walking meditation exercises.

I would occasionally take Spencer's entire group and practice meditation while walking. The group would go outside, and I would demonstrate how walking slowly, mindfully, erect, and deliberately could enhance meditation practice. I would discuss the importance of focus and breathing out with each step and breathing when lifting up. The group would start the meditation walk at one end of the yard, with me as the leader, and slowly walk to the other end, being mindful of each step. At the conclusion of the exercise the group discussed their experiences with each other. I would ask them how it felt to be walking slowly, the sensations in their bodies, and the emotions that might have surfaced. I suggested this method of meditation along with sitting meditations as options for practice.

I believe the combination of bringing the focus into the here and now, the breathing exercises, guided imagery, music, spirituality group, and identifying process in the moment all helped Spencer in his pursuit of continuous, meaningful sobriety. Spencer was also an accomplished drummer and found that regular practice on his drum kit was meditative. I encouraged him to use this as an additional method to enhance his meditative practices.

## Present Moment-Tao

I believe what I did with Spencer in counseling addressed what was already present. The use of imagery helped him identify a safe place within himself to relax and focus on feelings and positive affirmations. I did not incorporate spirituality into the sessions; rather it was present like the Tao. I worked with Spencer through his pained spirit as well as through his joy, and helped him understand that his joy was in relationship to the pain he had suffered most of his life, and to how he had survived. He also knew that in order to keep what he had obtained in recovery he needed to help others in pain.

I believe Spencer knew his days were numbered at our last session, having burnt the candle at both ends for over forty years. I spent time with him around the darkness that had befallen throughout his addiction, helped him see the importance of his own struggles, and how they would come again in different forms. I believe he understood how his life had arisen from the ashes and with each day he was given, he had an opportunity to be sober and present for his family, as well as a provider of support to others trying to get sober.

## Concluding Thoughts

To live a full spiritual life is to be actively involved in the present moment with our emotions, with our selves, and to genuinely accept where we are at that given moment. We can't change the past, nor can we predict the future. We can, however, live in today, one day at a time. Spirituality is not meant to be complicated; in fact, I believe simplicity is the key. I understood my limitations, my powerlessness, and my compassion when working with Spencer. I did not do anything; rather I was present, authentic, and willing to confront the process in the moment. In so doing, I felt I was helping him understand his own present reality and spirit. My interventions were humble attempts at exploring the spiritual realm of his recovery. How arrogant it would have been for me to believe that I had a clear understanding of how his spirituality worked. I tried instead to connect with his essence or spirit and provide in the therapeutic setting an atmosphere of acceptance and genuine compassion.

Spencer knew I would go to hell with him, but not for him. I would be with him on his journey, as much or as little as he desired. Most important, in working with all of my clients, is my ongoing commitment to personal growth, for in that parallel process is where our spirits touch.

### References
Alcoholics Anonymous. (1976). *Alcoholics Anonymous.* New York: AA World Services.

Gorski, T. (1989). *Passages through recovery: An action plan for preventing relapse.* Center City, MN: Hazelden.

Jung, C. G. (1974). *The Bill W.–Carl Jung letters.* A.A. Grapevine, Reprinted in A.A. Grapevine, 26–31.

Kurtz, E. (1979). *Not-God: A history of Alcoholics Anonymous.* Center City, MN: Hazelden.

Matthews, C. O. (1998). Integrating the spiritual dimension into traditional counselor education programs. *Counseling and Values, 43,* 3–18.

Tiebout, H. A. (1944). *Conversion as a psychological phenomenon.* New York: National Council on Alcoholism.

Wildish, P. (2000). *The book of Ch'I.* Boston: Tuttle Publishing.

Yalom, I. (1995). *The theory and practice of group psychotherapy* (4th ed.). New York: Basic Books.

# Seven Stages of Spiritual Development: A Framework to Solve Psycho-Spiritual Problems

## Daya Singh Sandhu

Spirituality is the highest good, the *summum bonum,* of human life. For this reason, I attach great importance to spirituality in my own life and in the lives of my clients. It is encouraging to note that at the cusp of the new millennium, the study of spirituality is rapidly gaining a great momentum, resurgence, and prominence in all fields in general, and in the helping professions in particular. Since discussion about the role of spirituality in counseling and psychotherapy is relatively new and the study of spirituality as a new field is just emerging, there seem to be many perspectives and few points of consensus. I feel this lack of consensus makes the study of spirituality rather more fascinating and intriguing than limiting or confusing. New perspectives give a renewed sense of freshness.

In this chapter, I present some of my own perspectives on spirituality based on my unique background in Eastern philosophy and Sikhism. First of all, I would like to define spirituality, discuss spiritual types, and focus on human problems. I will also propose seven stages of spirituality as an integral part of human development. This chapter will also present some discussion about the newly developed *Experience Based Spiritual Development Scale* (EBSDS) by Sandhu and Asrabadi (2003). A spiritual autobiography of a graduate student will be presented and interpreted to demonstrate application of my thoughts and perspectives on the role of spirituality in counseling and psychotherapy.[1]

## Definition of Spirituality

There is no general consensus about how to define spirituality. Because interest has increased in this subject, there is a large array of definitions. It seems that spirituality means different things to different people. There are as many definitions of spirituality as there are different individuals. For instance, Benner defined spirituality as "Our response to a deep and mysterious human yearning for self-transcendence and surrender, a yearning to find our place" (1989, p. 21). Holmes described it as "The human capacity for relationship with that which transcends sense phenomena" (1982, p. 12). I define spirituality as a conscious or unconscious human desire to search for the ultimate love or union with the Higher-Self through transcendence, compassion for others, reverence for life, and appreciation of nature. In short, I believe that spirituality is a *human yearning for divine love.* It is the very perpetual pain of the soul that longs for union with the Almighty or the Higher-Self.

In this chapter, I will focus on spirituality, not religion. I believe a religion may be a means, but spirituality is the end, the ultimate destination. I agree with Berenson when he distinguished between religion and spirituality stating, "Spirituality, as opposed to religion, connotes a direct, personal experience of the sacred, unmediated by particular belief systems prescribed by dogma or by hierarchical structures of priests, ministers, rabbis, or gurus" (1990, p. 59).

## Paths to Spirituality

While I reject the idea of classifying "spirituality," the different ways to become spiritual can be classified. For instance, when we talk about Christian spirituality, Islamic spirituality, or Buddhist spirituality, we are really talking about three different religions as three different pathways to spirituality. Spirituality remains the same, the relationship with God

---

[1] **Editor's Note:** This chapter presents Daya's own theory of spiritual development which underlies his approach and the construction of the EBSDS. I am grateful to him for sharing this material with us and for showing its application in a clinical case. Chapter Appendix A contains a copy of the EBSDS instrument. Appendix B lists some follow-up, open-ended questions.

or with the Higher-Self. To me the word *spirituality* is the most sacred word, and the relationship with the Supreme is the most valued, purest, and loftiest one.

There are three main sources for developing or getting in touch with our spirituality: scriptures, spiritual guides, and innate resources. *Scriptural* sources are any sacred or religious writing or books, *spiritual guides* are individuals who show the way such as a living guru or spiritual master, and *innate resources* are those allowing a person to become spiritual entirely through one's own thoughts and actions.

## Spirituality in Counseling and Psychotherapy

Unfortunately in the past, the spiritual dimension of human behavior has not been given the necessary significance it deserves in counseling and psychology. On the contrary, pioneering figures in psychology such as Sigmund Freud (1961) totally rejected religion and denounced it as pathological. He was convinced that people must abandon religion altogether if they would like to act more maturely. Also, for too long human experience has been presented as unidimensional (biological) or bidimensional (psycho-social). It was Engel who proposed three dimensions of human behavior in 1977, that is *bio-psycho-social.* It was only in 1999 that Wilber proposed five dimensions of human behavior: biological, psychological, social, moral, religious or spiritual.

I believe that human behavior is multidimensional (Sandhu & Aspy, 1997). Humans are not only psychosexual (Freud, 1933), or psychosocial (Erikson, 1963), but they are also psycho-spiritual, and I consider spirituality an essential dimension of human development. A person is not whole or holy without it. In addition to physical development, cognitive development, emotional development, moral development, and psychosocial development, it is imperative that mental health professionals place the necessary emphasis on their clients' spiritual development. To me, spiritual development is the *ultimate* human development.

### Spirituality as a Fifth Force in Counseling

The psychodynamic, behavioral, humanistic, and multicultural are generally identified as the four main forces in counseling and psychology (Essandoh, 1996). By "force" it is meant that each of these perspectives has widely impacted a variety of helping professions, such as counseling, psychology, social work, and nursing. They have also influenced other fields, including education and medicine. It must be noted that each of these "forces" is not only pervasive and potent, but also prevalent on a continuing basis.

Generally speaking, Abraham Maslow is credited with identifying and naming the first three forces: psychodynamics, behaviorism, and humanism. Multiculturalism was first named by Paul Pedersen (1991, 1999) as the fourth force. I suggest that spirituality should be identified as the *fifth force* (Sandhu, in press; Stanard, Sandhu & Painter, 2000). In spite of the assertions made by Pate and Bondi (1992) and Frame and Williams (1996) that spirituality is an offshoot of multiculturalism, I believe that spirituality itself is pancultural and overarching, and it can stand independently as the *fifth force* in counseling and psychology (Sandhu, in press).

Fortunately, the psycho-spiritual dimension is gaining recognition as a strong force in the view of human personality. There has been an increase in interest in spiritual matters, and this has been reflected in both popular and professional literatures in America (Richards & Bergin, 1997). The present book with nationally known authors and its editor, Dr. Oliver Morgan, is another example that reflects the *zeitgeist* of the new millennium.

It is clear that spiritual issues are also coming more into the focus of other disciplines such as medicine (e.g., Daaleman & Frey, 1999) and nursing (e.g, Narayanasamy, 1999) to name a few. Thomas (1999) reported an increase from 4 of 135 to 40 of 135 medical schools offering a course on religious and spiritual issues. Since 1996, psychiatric residency programs in the United States are required to formally address religious and spiritual issues in training (Brawer, Handal, Fabricatore, Roberts & Wajda-Johnston, 2002). The American Psychiatric Association (2000) includes "Religious or Spiritual Problem" as part of its section on "Other Conditions That May Be a Focus of Clinical Attention" (p. 313). Richards and Bergin (1997) asserted that the spirit of the times is ripe for bringing spirituality into mainstream theory and practice. Therefore, the recognition of spirituality as a *fifth force* can no longer be ignored or dismissed.

### Role of Spirituality in Human Problems

Human problems can be broadly classified into three main categories, namely problems of the body, the mind, and the soul or life force. In addition, the human mind is capable of affecting both the body and the soul, as illustrated in Figure 1.

We are already aware of so-called psychosomatic effects, when the mind affects the body negatively or positively. When the mind affects the soul, these problems become psycho-spiritual. Western psychology has already

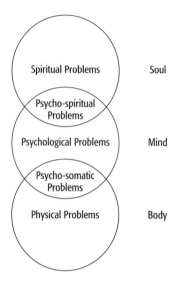

Spiritual Problems          Soul

Psycho-spiritual
Problems

Psychological Problems      Mind

Psycho-somatic
Problems

Physical Problems           Body

FIGURE 1    Body Mind Soul

placed significant emphasis on somatic, psychosomatic, and psychological problems, but the study of spiritual or psycho-spiritual problems is
relatively new.

## Ultimate Reasons for Human Problems

In the final analysis all psychological problems, properly understood, have
their origin in spiritual need. A person's feelings of guilt about a specific
issue—for example, feelings of guilt stemming from the perception of not
doing a good enough job to obtain a raise in pay—may reflect broader
feelings of guilt about not being good enough for life in general. I propose calling this *ultimate guilt,* as I would similarly recognize *ultimate
anxiety* and *ultimate fear,* as well as *ultimate love, ultimate development,* and *ultimate sacrifice.* An analysis of Ingersoll's (2001) *Spiritual Wellness Inventory*
can help demonstrate that "all problems are actually spiritual problems."
Ingersoll has proposed ten dimensions of his inventory including "Conception of the Absolute/Divine, Meaning, Connectedness, Mystery, Spiritual
Freedom, Experience/Ritual, Forgiveness, Hope, Knowledge/Learning,
and Present-Centeredness." This means that a person's problem can be
traced back or is connected in some way to a person's spiritual well-being.
For instance, without a feeling of connectedness a person would feel lonely,

depressed, and isolated. Without mystery, a person would have no faith in life after death and a sense of *ultimate anxiety* may prevail. If a person does not possess the ability to forgive, then he or she would always feel guilt, remorse, and anger. While it is not possible to discuss all ten dimensions here, it must be noted that when one spiritual dimension is in distress all others also suffer.

## Seven Stages of Spirituality

Frame (2003) discussed the work of five theorists who focused on the linear or hierarchical progress of people's religious or faith development. These theorists included Gordon Allport's (1950) Theory of Religious Sentiments, James Fowler's (1981) Stages of Faith Development, Michael Washburn's (1988) Stages of Psychospiritual Development, Fritz Oser's (1991) Stages of Religious Judgment, and Genia's (1995) Stages of Faith. All these models are useful for counselors and psychotherapists because they provide a framework for understanding how clients develop religious or spiritual interests. These models also help counselors identify the critical transitional points where intervention strategies become imperative.

I have three major criticisms of these models, however. First, I don't believe that spiritual development necessarily progresses in a linear fashion or in sequential stages as suggested in these models. I believe that spiritual maturity develops in a desultory manner. Second, most of these models seem to mirror Kohlberg's stages of Moral Development or Piaget's Cognitive Development Stages (Gathman & Nessan, 1997). Since "experiencing is believing" in spirituality, I would argue for spiritual development being based more on social learning theory. Third, these models have confounded spirituality with religion. Spirituality and religion are presented as intertwined. I consider religion as a means to spirituality and thus they need to be discussed separately.

I conceptualized the following seven experiential stages of spirituality. Religion may or may not play a role in them. I think of these stages as the *experience-based stages of spirituality* (Sandhu & Asrabadi, 2003). These stages are briefly introduced here.

### Experience Based Stages of Spiritual Development

1. *Scourge.* This is a stage which can best be described as "a-spiritual," or a stage when a person's spiritual interests are dormant. At this level, the individual is mostly egocentric and is focused only on materialistic matters. Spirituality is of very little or no interest. I call life without spiritual awakening, *a scourge.*

*2. Emerge.* In some cases, *emerging* from the previous stage of *scourge* results from a major life event or trauma, which leads a person to become spiritual. It seems that in a time of crisis, all humans become spiritual and/or religious. In other cases, an awakening to spiritual life might be facilitated by a spiritual teacher, a preceptor, or a guru. Of course, a guru could be any person who removes our spiritual darkness or ignorance and introduces us to the spiritual realm. In the absence of a living guru, a scripture can serve as the source of inspiration. This stage can be described as a transforming stage and can also be conducive to transitioning to higher stages. Spirituality becomes important for a person for the first time during this stage. A person takes deliberate interest in it.

*3. Purge.* The *purge* stage is characterized by an individual's rejecting materialistic and worldly pleasures. At this level the individual changes path. Spiritual concerns become more important than materialistic interests. A part of the purging process may include turning away from a life of scourge. A person makes a conscious effort to curtail or manage several deadly habits, such as lust, anger, greed, worldly attachments, and haughtiness, since these are the barriers to spiritual life.

*4. Diverge.* Spiritual ascent is not steady or linear. A person might start experiencing *divergence,* leaving a spiritual path and going back to old materialistic ways of living. There may be a loss of interest in spiritual matters during this stage. This setback is generally transitory.

*5. Resurge.* During the *resurgence* stage individuals are coming back to a stronger spiritual understanding after having "slipped," regressed, or suffered a loss of interest in a previous spiritual journey. This spiritual understanding and interest is stronger than previous experiences. At this stage, spirituality and/or religion become important once again. One's interest in spirituality is revived or renewed even more vigorously.

*6. Converge.* Persons experiencing *convergence* are really on a very deliberate and conscious spiritual path. Their spiritual beliefs, spiritual feelings, and spiritual actions are all in synchrony. A spiritual person starts living his or her life proactively according to the special rules for living as required by the scriptures or by high moral and spiritual standards. At this level, a person experiences greater solace and satisfaction by balancing spiritual and materialistic matters. Clearly, there is comfort in walking on this path where there is faith, hope, and an appreciation for life.

*7. Merge.* I believe that the *merge* stage is the ultimate in spiritual development. There is emphasis on experience of union with God or Oneness. This stage also has mystical qualities. This stage is characterized with one uniting with a Higher Being. Life and death are both blessings.

At this highest stage of spiritual realization, suffering and comforts are the same as they both come from the same Higher-Self or the Supreme Being. A person generally achieves the highest level of serenity at this stage.

## Assessing Spirituality

A person's "stage" or "moment" on the spiritual journey can be identified by using the "Experience Based Spiritual Development Scale (EBSDS)" developed and empirically tested by Sandhu and Asrabadi (2003). It must be noted that all persons have psychological or psycho-spiritual concerns at each of these stages, especially at the critical transition points. For instance, a sense of meaninglessness or spiritual emptiness will generally be prevalent at the scourge stage. A sense of spiritual emergency and depression are felt at the emergence stage. Leaving old behaviors and adopting a new spiritually oriented life style could be quite stressful. While diverging, it is but natural to feel guilty. Resurgence could create some ambivalent feelings. The last two stages, "converge" and "merge" could create separation anxiety, caused by the drift from the material world to the spiritual realm.

Counselors are encouraged to use this scale, EBSDS, to determine the current spiritual stage/s at which their clients are functioning. They could also help their clients prepare a psycho-spiritual profile to determine their counseling or psychological needs. Based on their needs, counselors must provide psychological or psycho-spiritual help as warranted.

## Goals of Psycho-Spiritual Counseling and Therapy

I consider spiritual development as the *ultimate development*. For this reason, the basic purpose of counseling and psychotherapy is to help clients become more spiritually developed or awakened. Therapy may enhance clients' awareness and help them take significant steps for the edification of their souls to achieve transcendence and intimacy. As a matter of fact, therapy can become a spiritual process itself (Benner, 1989).

*Care* of the soul and *cure* of the soul are two additional important concepts that should be of great interest to counselors and psychotherapists. According to Moore (1992), we have to learn the task of organizing and shaping our lives for the good of the soul. According to Szasz, cure of the soul "is closely linked to a number of basic concepts, such as wrongdoing, guilt, repentance, confession, conversion, and change of mind" (1978, p. 32). Interestingly, all these concepts are also the major concerns of counseling, psychology, and psychotherapy.

Furthermore, from my own perspective, the ultimate goal of spiritual counseling and psychotherapy is to help clients develop a sense of *serenity* or a sense of equanimity. This is the dimension of spiritual development when people lose the sense of duality or black-and-white thinking. It is also the highest stage of faith when a person has all faith and no doubts. Benner (1989) describes it as the integration of action and thought, conscious and unconscious, interior life and external behavior, and body and soul. I believe that serenity or equanimity is a condition when a person's heart becomes like a deep ocean. In this deep ocean, the waves and turbulence of sorrows and troubles come and go, but the deep ocean stays the same, just calm.

## A Case Example

With written permission, the following spiritual autobiography of Carolyn Sisk is reproduced here. Carolyn was also asked to complete the *Experience Based Spiritual Development Scale* (EBSDS). The results and related discussion follows her biographical account.

---

## MY SPIRITUAL JOURNEY:
### An Autobiographical Account

#### Carolyn Sisk

I was born in rural Tennessee on my maternal grandparents' property. My father was a farmer and my mother was a homemaker. I had one brother two years older. I was born on Friday the 13th and my mother has always said it was a lucky day for them because they wanted a daughter. My parents were Christians and my early history consisted of sporadic attendance at small country churches. I remember no specific rituals or specific talk about religion or spirituality.

When I was in first grade, my parents moved to Detroit so my father could make a better living for his family. We started attending a full gospel church when I was about eight. My parents felt comfortable in that church because the congregation and leaders were people from the south and many were from close to where we lived in Tennessee. The people were wonderful and caring. I established close friendships with people of my own age. My social activities were centered on the church and my relatives that lived in the Detroit area.

It was at this small Pentecostal Holiness Church that I first professed my belief in Jesus Christ as my personal savior and I became a member of the church. There were many strict rules. Make-up, movies, dancing, and dating outside the "faith" were sins and would put a person in danger of "burning in the lake of fire if I was called home before repenting." It was a struggle to stay in the confines of the rules and be a teenager that wanted to be popular and have fun. People could "backslide" or fall out of the grace of God for doing evil. I felt as if I was always asking for forgiveness and then doing something wrong and then I would have to pray my way back into the fold. Nevertheless, I had moments of divine communion with God. I was also emotionally involved with God. Certain songs, sermons, prayers, and testimonies could kindle the flame and I would be praising God with songs and prayer. I cherish my memories of the fine people and wonderful experiences I had at that small church in Detroit. It was the religion of my parents and it gave me a strong foundation to build on as I continued my journey.

I sporadically attended church when I went away to college. I met my future husband when I was a freshman and our lives centered on sorority and fraternity activities. I did attend my church when I would go home for the holidays and summer. When I was a sophomore, a significant experience happened when I was home. I was praying and I received a premonition that I would be in a car accident. I prayed I would be safe. The accident happened when I was driving in Montgomery, Alabama. An elderly lady ran a red light and hit us broadside, but everyone escaped unharmed.

After college I married and we moved to Pittsburgh. Church was not a priority. Being married was hard work. I had been married four years when I was diagnosed with cancer. I had extensive surgery to eradicate the cancer. It was a frightening time in my life. I said many prayers and others prayed for me. My prettiest aunt came to be with my mother during my surgery. I remember being in terrible pain after the surgery. My aunt sat beside me and stroked my arm and hand. Suddenly, the pain subsided and I felt a great calmness. She said, "I prayed for the pain to go away." As I was recovering, my father made a profound statement of faith.

Crying, he told me that he had resolved that he "would not go back on God even if the cancer took my life." That resolve to stand with God in times of crises has been very important to me.

My prognosis was uncertain and the doctor said I must not have children for five years or more. I was devastated because the gynecologist had given me a diagnosis of endometriosis and he said it would be difficult for me to have children and gradually I would become infertile and then sterile. I felt very sad but miracles do happen. In a few months I discovered I was pregnant. I was elated because I had always dreamed of having children. Still there was the nagging possibility that I might be putting myself at great risk and the baby also. The dichotomy of elation and despair began to overwhelm me. One day when I was about eight months pregnant I was standing in the shower and I was overcome with the thought that I might die and not be able to raise my baby. I started crying and praying until I completely surrendered my future, my life, and my baby's life to God. I confessed that I couldn't continue to carry the burden of uncertainty and that I was turning everything over to God. My allegiance was with God and EVERYTHING was in His hands. The most wonderful sense of peace overcame me. Words cannot describe the absolute peace that I felt. When I became pregnant with our son and as the years wore on, there were times that the worry crept back but I could reach back and feel that wonderful peace and know that I was in God's hands and that the future was also in His hands.

We moved to Atlanta and then to Cincinnati. When our two children started school, we started going to church again. I was baptized but it was not a significant spiritual experience for me. When we moved to Louisville, we found a wonderful church to join. We made many friends and shared many experiences with the members. I always have a wonderful peaceful feeling when I walk up to the doors of my church. We took our children to church and they participated in many youth activities. But life became more difficult when our children became teenagers. Our daughter challenged us with some of her behavior, but she has grown into a beautiful adult and friend. I cherish her.

Our son began experimenting with drugs and became addicted. He followed the Grateful Dead for months at a time. There were long stretches of time when I didn't know where he was or if he was alive. Many prayers went up for him. He tried to quit. We had interventions with him twice and the last time he entered a rehab

program himself. My second significant spiritual experience occurred when I was especially grieved and worried. I knelt by my
bed and prayed a prayer of complete surrender to God's will. I felt
that I could not walk another step with such grief over my son's
choices. I literally held my hand up to God and said, "He's yours.
You love him more than me. Take him. I trust you, God, even if
he dies." This giving up my control over my son's behavior saved
my sanity. I didn't stop praying or welcoming him home or loving
his hugs and the talks we had. I would pray for the right words to
say to him that would make a difference. I read books and got
counseling. I told him I had learned more from him than anyone
in my life.

On September 2, 2001, I found my son's body on the floor of
the downstairs bathroom. He died of an overdose. He was 26 years
old. He had been in recovery for over seven months before he
started using again. His sponsor approached me crying at my son's
funeral. He said he was so sorry and that he should have done
more. At first I didn't know what to say, but then God gave me a
beautiful thought. I told him my son's sobriety for the past months
was the most wonderful gift I have ever received. We had talked
of many things spiritual and mundane. It's a terrible thing to lose
a child. He was a gift. I told both of my children many times that
they were gifts from God because of the circumstances of their
births after my cancer surgery. I also remember my father's words
about still trusting God no matter what our circumstances.

God has been with me through it all. I continue to pray and
ask God to keep my faith strong and to give me peace. I feel I have
a special commission to help addicts. I have some tentative plans
that need to be developed more fully. Others helped my son and
now it's time for me to help.

## Critical Analysis or Interpretation of Carolyn's Spiritual Autobiography

My graduate assistant, Scott Berry, a doctoral candidate in Counseling
Psychology, interpreted Carolyn's spiritual autobiography from the
perspective of my proposed seven stages of spirituality. Here is Scott's
critical analysis.

Several elements of the proposed seven stages of spirituality are illustrated in Carolyn's spiritual autobiography. Early in Carolyn's life, there

were some aspects of *Scourge* operating. As a child, she knew her parents were Christians, she attended church sporadically, and recalls no specific discussions or activities related to religion or spirituality. There is little evidence in her account of these early years of the beginnings of her spiritual awakening.

When Carolyn was in first grade and she moved to Detroit and started attending a full Gospel church, one can see the qualities associated with the stage of *Emergence*. The move and attendance at church were clearly major life events, which lead her to become more spiritual in her approach to life.

The author's struggles as a teenager had elements of both *Emergence* and *Divergence*. As a teenager, she had some special experiences in her relationship to God, which is associated with *Emergence*. She was torn by the pressures of being a teenager, which likely resulted in losing some interest in living a spiritual life, or *Diverging*.

When Carolyn attended college, she clearly experienced some *Divergence*, but still had some spiritual moments consistent with *Emerge*. Her prayer and premonition would seem to have qualities of *Emergence*, since her car accident was a major life event that kept her somewhat spiritually attuned.

As the author married, she continued in her *Divergence* stage. After diagnosis of cancer, its treatment, and pregnancy, her focus on relationship with God and spirituality increased tremendously. She experienced elements of *Purge*. She began to become more spiritually focused and also experienced *Resurgence* as she gained an understanding of her spiritual journey. This part of her life was clearly marked by a stronger sense of spirituality than at any other point in her life up until that point.

Carolyn's *Resurgence* continued when her family made a few moves. When her children started school, she began attending church and eventually found a great church in Louisville. She began to show signs of *Convergence*, evidenced by the peace and happiness she experienced during this time.

She experienced her most progressive spiritual stage during the time her son battled drug addiction. She experienced *Merge* in her relationship to God, especially regarding her son's drug problem. It seems that she felt a union with God. Her prayer life and concern for others were strong. This time in her life also had some qualities of the *Emerge* stage as a major life trauma pushed her spiritual development along.

Some time after her son's death, Carolyn seemed very much at peace. She also had a strong sense of union with God and was experiencing *Merge*. Her continued focus on her spiritual life and helping others shows how Carolyn has achieved much in her spiritual development, moving from a personal to transpersonal level.

## Administration and Interpretation of Carolyn's EBSDS Results

The newly developed *Experience Based Spiritual Development Scale* (2003) was administered to Carolyn to determine her spiritual development stage. Carolyn's percentile scores on the subscales of EBSDS resulted as follows:

1. Scourge: 16. 67%
2. Emerge: 95. 24%
3. Purge: 80. 66%
4. Diverge: 33. 33%
5. Resurge: 85. 71%
6. Converge: 96. 66%
7. Merge: 50. 00%

**Interpretations of Percentile Scores** When compared to materialistic matters, Carolyn's spiritual interests outweigh them significantly. She is now awakened spiritually. In order to lead a spiritual life, she had curtailed, shunned, or eliminated those behaviors that are considered mundane or worldly in nature. She lived a life that follows religious and spiritual laws. After losing interest in spiritual matters for a while, her spiritual interests have resurged with greater zeal and intensity. Carolyn also made deliberate or proactive efforts to gain spiritual knowledge, and her daily activities are full of spiritual enthusiasm. She appears in sync with the Higher-Self, and there is little disparity between her daily life and expected spiritual or religious commandments. She seems to be at peace with the Supreme. In worldly matters, she has moved from personal to transpersonal in her efforts to help the addicted.

## Carolyn's Answers to Open Ended Questions

In addition to administration of the *Experience Based Spiritual Development Scale,* Carolyn was asked to respond to open-ended questions listed in Appendix B. These questions were divided into two groups. The first group of questions was for those people who considered themselves spiritual; the second group of questions was designed for those people who have little or no interest in spiritual matters. As Carolyn considers herself a very spiritual person, her answers to fifteen questions follow. The purpose of these open-ended questions was to complement or supplement Carolyn's information to prepare her psycho-spiritual profile.

**Directions:** How would you describe yourself?

A. A spiritual person
B. A person with little or no interest in spiritual matters

If you consider yourself a spiritual person or a person with strong interests in spirituality, please answer questions under part A. If not, please answer questions under part B. Please limit your answers to two to three paragraphs.

### Part A: A Person with Spiritual Interests

1. *Is spirituality important to you and why?*

   Peace, acceptance, and living in the moment are gifts that I experience when I am feeling close to God. These gifts are priceless and help me to cope with difficult circumstances.

2. *What are some of your spiritual beliefs?*

   • God is all knowing and all powerful.

   • I have done nothing to earn God's love—it is given. It is grace.

   • God knew me while I was still in the womb and I am so important to him that He knows the number of hairs on my head.

   • Life is a journey between eternities and some day I will be with the people I love and who have died and have gone to live with God.

3. *How do you practice or put spirituality in your daily life?*

   I pray often. I try to treat others with respect. I try to examine motives for my actions. I repent for things that I know to be wrong. I try not to judge others for their actions. We're all trying to do the best we can with the knowledge we have so I forgive others. I am God's missionary and I want people to see God in me and in my behavior.

4. *When did you start taking interest in spirituality deliberately?*

   When I was about 12 years old.

5. *What specific incident/s do you recall which turned your life around to make you a spiritual person?*

   It's a continuous process. Specific people who invited me to be a Christian and taught me how to confess and ask forgiveness. Having cancer at 26 years and putting my future in God's hands. A group of 7 women from my church who helped me when things were difficult in my personal life. My son's death at 26 and my daughter's diagnosis of MS at age 26.

6. *How would you describe your relationship with God or the Higher-Self?*

   I am confident that I am loved beyond measure. I am undeserving but His grace is sufficient in all circumstances.

7. *To whom do you turn for help and hope when you are in deep trouble?*

   I turn to God, my friends, and family. Sometimes I try to work it out myself but Life has taught me that I don't have the answers. "We see through a glass darkly."

8. *Who is your ultimate source of power? Who would you call upon for strength or special help?*

   Family, friends, but ultimately it is God.

9. *How are your spiritual or religious beliefs helpful to you?*

   In my darkest hours of despair.

10. *What is the most meaningful or important thing in your life?*

    God.

11. *Was there any major life event or trauma in your life which led you to become increasingly more interested in spirituality?*

    Yes, there have been several. See question number 5.

12. *After changing path to spirituality, are there any behaviors that you had to curtail, shun, or stop?*

    I'm still a work in process. I've never been a really bad person. I am more aware of my behavior and motives now.

13. *After loss of interest in spiritual matters for some time, I am coming back with greater enthusiasm by engaging in many new behaviors such as:*

    I'm starting in a new group at my church called "Companions in Christ," which will meet for two hours on Sunday for about ten months.

14. *I live my life in accordance with religious or spiritual laws. For instance,*

    I attend religious services, I have standards for my behavior, I read the scripture, and I pray often.

15. *I feel that I am in sync with the Higher Being, which makes me feel . . .*

    That I am loved beyond measure.

### Preparation of Carolyn's Psycho-spiritual Profile

Carolyn's psycho-spiritual profile reflects someone whose thoughts, beliefs, actions, and feelings are representative of a spiritually mature person. Clearly Carolyn professed her spiritual beliefs in the Bible and Christianity when she wrote in response to Question No. 2, "I have done nothing to earn God's love—it is given. It is grace." Furthermore, "God knew me while I was still in the womb and I am so important to Him that He knows the number of hairs on my head" are reminiscent of lines from the Bible. Carolyn's answer to Question No. 3 explains that all her feelings, actions, and thoughts are imbued with spirituality. She seems to have moved from the mundane world and is longing to enter more fully into the spiritual sphere of her life. Standing at the threshold of the spiritual world, she declared, "I am God's missionary and I want people to see God in me and in my behavior."

From many major life events and traumas of her life, Carolyn has learned that there are no easy answers. Ultimately all answers are in His hands. Carolyn is in the process of completing a spiritual transformation, a phenomenon called *Jivan Mukt* in Hindu scriptures. A person called *Jivan Mukat,* or "freed from bondage," experiences spiritual salvation while still living in a human body.

## Integration of Spiritual Intervention Strategies

It is important that mental health professionals understand the goals of their therapeutic interventions. If clients bring spiritual issues into the counseling session, we must address them by integrating them with the traditional approaches. However, if spiritual issues are not important to clients, we must not encroach upon this territory to impose our spiritual views and beliefs on our clients. As suggested by Matthews (1998, p. 274), as a part of the intake information, a counselor might ask questions such as those stated below to find out a client's interest in religious or spiritual matters.

1. Is religion or spirituality important to you?
2. Do your religious or spiritual beliefs influence the way you look at your problems and the way you think about your health?
3. Would you like me to address your religious or spiritual beliefs and practices with you?

If a client is interested in discussing spiritual issues, some additional information can be obtained by using questions listed in Appendix B.

As mental health professionals, we are there to help clients with their spiritual issues, but we should not impose our views upon them if they are not ready or willing to discuss spiritual matters. We must understand our professional boundary and leave the evangelical wishes to priests, gurus, bhais, kazis, rabbis, and imams.

It is quite evident from Carolyn's autobiographical account and intake information that spirituality is extremely important to her. It has been a source of healing for her in dealing with cancer, endometriosis, her desire to have children, her son's drug addiction, and finally his death from a drug overdose. Amid all the overwhelming problems of life, Carolyn surrendered herself to God to find solace, peace of mind, and serenity when she wrote, "I started crying and praying until I completely surrendered my future, my life, and my baby's life to God. I confessed that I couldn't continue to carry the burden of uncertainty and that I was turning everything over to God. My allegiance was with God and EVERYTHING was in His hands. The most wonderful sense of peace overcame me. Words cannot express the absolute peace that I felt."

To work with Carolyn, a therapist might use three phases of counseling, as described by Len Sperry (2001). In phase one, a counselor must establish a therapeutic or working alliance with her by creating trust, hope, and faith. A therapist should also determine Carolyn's expectations from therapy and her readiness to focus on psycho-spiritual issues.

I believe that counselors in this phase would benefit from using Rogers's (1957) three facilitating conditions of empathy, congruence, and unconditional positive regard to build a good rapport with Carolyn. To integrate a spiritual perspective, I propose to add the word *transcendental* to these core conditions, suggesting that a counselor must have spiritual sensitivities to address Carolyn's psycho-spiritual problems.

Thus, *transcendental empathy* would mean that a counselor is able to view the client's world, from his or her own frame of reference, with a special attention to client's interest or concerns relating to religion and spirituality. Similarly, *transcendental congruence* and *transcendental unconditional positive regard* would mean that a client's religious or spiritual matters are given special attention by the counselor and these matters don't become a barrier in building a rapport with the client.

To integrate spirituality into counseling adequately, spirituality has to be considered at every step of the counseling process. For instance, even listening, the very basic and first step, will be changed to transcendental listening. *Transcendental listening* would mean that a counselor pays special attention to each client's language usage of religious or spiritual words, quotes, and messages. For instance, Carolyn's spiritual autobiography is replete with words and lines alluding to the Bible—clear evidence of the significance of spirituality in her life.

It is quite obvious from Carolyn's case example that overlooking the significance of religious or spiritual matters is missing a major dimension of clients' lives. I will go to the extent of asserting that omission of spiritual matters in counseling is unethical and underserves the clients.

Sperry's (2001) second phase warrants a comprehensive assessment. In addition to all other factors such as biological, sociological, and psychological, it is imperative that religious and spiritual factors also be considered as integral components of total assessment. The administration of the *Experience Based Spiritual Development Scale* (2003) could be helpful to determine and enhance the process of Carolyn's psycho-spiritual growth.

Carolyn's two highest percentile scores on EBSDS placed her clearly on two stages, *Emerge* and *Converge*. Her heart is awakened to spirituality and currently she is passing through a stage of *convergence*. As is characteristic of the convergence stage, Carolyn is really on her spiritual path. Her beliefs, spiritual feelings, and spiritual actions are all in synchronic relationship. Carolyn's answers to the open-ended question, *"How do you practice or put spirituality in your daily life?"* further corroborate this observation.

As stated earlier, when a person reaches the *Converge* stage he or she also starts living his or her life according to the special rules for living as required by the scriptures or by high moral and spiritual standards. At this level, a person experiences a great solace and satisfaction by balancing spiritual and materialistic matters. Clearly, there is a comfort in walking on this path where there is faith, hope, and an appreciation for life. These qualities are characteristic of Carolyn's current life style. At this *Converge* stage, a counselor can validate Carolyn's feelings and beliefs in order to support and guide her future spiritual explorations and endeavors.

In the third phase, "Planning and Implementing a Therapeutic Strategy," Sperry (2001, p. 16) recommends that spiritual counseling should focus on "implementing a strategy of healing, growth, and development." Various spiritual psychotherapeutic methods and spiritual interventions can be used to promote a client's healing and spiritual development depending on her stage of spiritual development. Faiver, Ingersoll, O'Brien, and McNally (2001) have suggested many specific interventions such as confessing, forgiving, praying, guiding, ritualizing, supporting, and so on that can be used very effectively at Carolyn's stage. She may also benefit from spiritual bibliotherapy and spiritually oriented counseling or psychotherapy groups.

Clearly, Carolyn has been in therapy for some time. As a graduate student, she is also very knowledgeable about the counseling field. She is well read and apparently she has reached the stage of self-acceptance and serenity. However, she still can benefit from spiritual counseling, in which a counselor can use traditional counseling theories and techniques with major or intentional focus on spirituality. For instance, while using a guided fantasy technique, the counselor can ask Carolyn to leave her problems with the Higher Power, God, or Jesus Christ. A counselor can pray with her or even teach her spiritual meditation. Carolyn might also use the counselor's help to make her plans to help addicts a reality.

## Concluding Thoughts

I would like to conclude this chapter with a suggestion that the spiritual transformation of our clients must transcend their own personal interests. Spiritually sublime or elevated persons must devote their spiritual energies to the welfare of others, their community, or the world, through their selfless service and sacrifice. A spiritual quietude generally ends in an incomplete journey. Carolyn's desire to help addicts as a special commission reflects such a resolve.

Lastly, we need to go beyond the narrow and rigid confines of the institutionalized religions. A spiritual path should be our ultimate path. Otherwise, there is a real danger that the religious flames now burning at the cusp of the new millennium will engulf us all. Only Truth can free us all, said Guru Nanak, as translated by Dr. Gopal Singh:

> There are many dogmas,
> There are many systems.
> There are many spiritual revelations
>
> Truth is above all these,
> But even higher is life lived in Truth.
> One Potter has fashioned all the pots,
> One Light pervades all creation.
> —Singh, 1978, p. 970

## References

Allport, G. W. (1950). *The individual and his religion.* New York: Macmillan.

American Psychiatric Association. (2000). *Desk reference to the diagnostic criteria from DSM-IV-TR.* Washington, DC: Author.

American Psychiatric Association. (2000). *Diagnostic and statistical manual of mental disorders: DSM-IV-TR.* Washington, DC: Author.

Barret, D. G. (1996). Religion: World religious statistics. In *Encyclopedia Britannica Book of the Year* (p. 298). Chicago, IL: Encyclopedia Britannica.

Benner, D. (1989). Toward a psychology of spirituality: Implications for personality and psychotherapy. *Journal of Psychology and Theology, 8,* 19–30.

Berenson, D. (1990). A systematic view of spirituality: God and Twelve Step programs as resources in family therapy. *Journal of Strategic and Systemic Therapies, 9,* 59–70.

Brawer, P. A., Handal, P. J., Fabricatore, A. N., Roberts, R., & Wajda-Johnson, V. A. (2002). Training and education in religion/spirituality with APA-accredited clinical psychology programs. *Professional Psychology: Research and Practice, 33,* 203–206.

Daaleman, T. P., & Frey, B. (1999). Spiritual and religious beliefs and practices of family physicians: A national survey. *Journal of Family Practice, 48,* 98–104.

Engel, G. (1977). The need for a new medical model: A challenge to biomedical science. *Science, 196,* 129–136.

Erikson, E. H. (1963). *Childhood and society* (2nd ed.). New York: Norton.

Essandoh, P. K. (1996). Multicultural counseling as the "fourth force": A call to arms. *Counseling Psychologist, 24*(1), 126–137.

Faiver, C., Ingersoll, R. E., O'Brien, E., & McNally, C. (2001). *Explorations in counseling and psychotherapy: Philosophical, practical, and personal reflections.* Belmont, CA: Brooks/Cole.

Fowler, J. W. (1981). *Stages of faith.* New York: Harper & Row.

Frame, M. W. (2003). *Integrating religion and spirituality into counseling.* Pacific Grove, CA: Brooks/ Cole.

Frame, M. W., & Williams, C. B. (1996). Counseling African Americans: Integrating spirituality in therapy. *Counseling and Values, 41,* 16–28.

Freud, S. (1961). The future of an illusion. In J. Strachey (Ed. and Trans.), *The standard edition of the complete psychological works of Sigmund Freud* (Vol. 21, pp. 1–56). London: Hogarth Press and the Institute of Psychoanalysis. (Original work published 1927.)

Freud, S. (1933). *New introductory lectures on psycho-analysis* (translated by W. H. J. Sprott). New York: W. W. Norton & Company.

Gathman, A. C., & Nessan, C. L. (1997). Fowler's stages of faith development in honors science and religion seminar. *Zygon, 32,* 407–414.

Genia, V. (1995). *Counseling and psychotherapy of religious clients: A developmental approach.* Westport, CT: Praeger.

Holmes, U. T. (1982). *Spirituality for ministry.* San Francisco: Harper & Row.

Ingersoll, E. (2001). The Spiritual Wellness Inventory. In C. Faiver, R. Ingersoll, E. O. Brien, and C. McNally, *Explorations in counseling and spirituality: Philosophical, practical, and personal reflections* (pp. 185–194). Belmont, CA: Wadsworth/Thomson Learning.

Matthews, D. (1998). *The faith factor: Proof of the healing power of prayer.* New York: Viking.

Moore, T. (1992). *Care of the soul: A guide for cultivating depth and sacredness in everyday life.* New York, NY: HarperCollins.

Narayanasamy, A. (1999). A review of spirituality as applied to nursing. *International Journal of Nursing Studies, 36,* 117–125.

Oser, F. K. (1991). The development of religious judgment. In F. K. Oser & W. G. Scarlett (Eds.), *Religious development in childhood and adolescence* (pp. 5–25). San Francisco: Jossey-Bass.

Pate, R. H., & Bondi, A. M. (1992). Religious beliefs and practice: An integral aspect of multicultural awareness. *Counselor Education and Supervision, 32,* 108–115.

Pedersen, P. (1991). Multiculturalism as a generic approach to counseling. *Journal of Counseling and Development, 70*(1), 6–12.

Pedersen, P. (1999). *Multiculturalism as a fourth force.* Philadelphia: Brunner/Mazel.

Richards, P. S., & Bergin, A. E. (1997). *A spiritual strategy for counseling and psychotherapy.* Washington, DC: American Psychological Association.

Rogers, C. (1957). The necessary and sufficient conditions of therapeutic personality change. *Journal of Consulting Psychology, 21,* 95–103.

Sandhu, D. S. (Ed.). (in press). *Spirituality as a fifth force in counseling: Implications for practice, research, and training.* Alexandria, VA: American Counseling Association.

Sandhu, D. S., & Aspy, C. B. (1997). *Counseling for prejudice prevention and reduction.* Alexandria, VA: American Counseling Association.

Sandhu, D. S., & Asrabadi, B. R. (2003). *Development of Experienced Based Spiritual Development Scale (EBSDS): Some preliminary findings.* Unpublished manuscript. University of Louisville, Louisville, KY.

Singh, G. (1978) (Translator). *Sri Guru Granth Sahib: English version.* Chandigarh, India: World Sikh University Press.

Sperry, L. (2001). *Spirituality in clinical practice: Incorporating the spiritual dimension in psychotherapy and counseling.* Philadelphia: Brunner-Routledge.

Stanard, R. P., Sandhu, D. S., & Painter, L. C. (2000). Assessment of spirituality in counseling. *Journal of Counseling & Development, 78*(2), 204–210.

Szasz. T. S. (1978). *The myth of psychotherapy: Mental healing as religion, rhetoric, and repression.* Garden City, NY: Anchor Press/Double Day.

Thomas, J. (1999). Psychotherapy and religion: Do they mix and blend? *National Psychologist (8),* 4–5.

Washburn, M. (1988). *The ego and the dynamic ground.* Albany, NY: State University of New York Press.

Wilber, K. (1999). *One taste: The journals of Ken Wilber.* Boston: Shambhala.

ॐ

# Experience Based Spiritual Development Scale (2003)

## Daya Singh Sandhu and Badiolah R. Asrabadi

**Directions:**   This scale is designed to determine the spiritual stage you are currently passing through. There are no right or wrong answers, but for the data to be meaningful, please answers all the questions the best you can. You may also feel free to substitute the words "Higher Power" in place of God, if you prefer.

*Please rate your responses on these statements as follows:*

| | |
|---|---|
| Strongly Disagree | 1 |
| Disagree | 2 |
| Moderately Disagree | 3 |
| Moderately Agree | 4 |
| Agree | 5 |
| Strongly Agree | 6 |

1. I am convinced that God cares
   for me.                        1   2   3   4   5   6

2. I believe that I am a vital instrument of a Higher Power for some
   purpose.                       1   2   3   4   5   6

3. I am turning more and more
   to God.                        1   2   3   4   5   6

4. I am transforming from a material-
   istic being to a spiritual being.    1    2    3    4    5    6

5. I often return to my former lifestyle when I am out of connection
   with my Higher Power.    1    2    3    4    5    6

6. I dwell with God all the time,
   experiencing complete peace.    1    2    3    4    5    6

7. I don't derive much satisfaction
   from spiritual matters.    1    2    3    4    5    6

8. I have experienced God's presence.    1    2    3    4    5    6

9. I help others with their spiritual
   concerns.    1    2    3    4    5    6

10. More and more, I believe in the
    existence of God.    1    2    3    4    5    6

11. I deeply value my relationship
    with God.    1    2    3    4    5    6

12. I believe that God is everywhere
    at all times.    1    2    3    4    5    6

13. Compared to materialistic inter-
    ests, I am getting more and more
    interested in spiritual matters.    1    2    3    4    5    6

14. I am returning to God with
    deeper conviction.    1    2    3    4    5    6

15. I believe in God, but there have
    been times when I have not
    respected or worshipped Him.    1    2    3    4    5    6

16. I am now able to spiritually
    accept my Higher Power leading
    and guiding my life.    1    2    3    4    5    6

17. I consider prayer to be just a
    waste of time.                          1    2    3    4    5    6

18. By God's grace, all things are
    possible.                               1    2    3    4    5    6

19. There is a Higher Power who
    loves all.                              1    2    3    4    5    6

20. I regularly participate in
    activities that are necessary to
    enhance my spirituality.                1    2    3    4    5    6

21. I am beginning to find that my
    life has a purpose.                     1    2    3    4    5    6

22. I am more determined now that
    spirituality is the right path for me.  1    2    3    4    5    6

23. I have not been able to consistently
    sustain my spiritual behaviors.         1    2    3    4    5    6

24. I no longer care about the
    concerns of the material world,
    only of my spirituality.                1    2    3    4    5    6

25. I have no interest in spiritual
    matters.                                1    2    3    4    5    6

26. Prayers are very satisfying to
    me spiritually.                         1    2    3    4    5    6

27. My faith in God has helped me
    to cope with the difficult times
    in my life.                             1    2    3    4    5    6

28. I feel one with God and the
    universe.                               1    2    3    4    5    6

29. God is my personal guide and
    a helper.                               1    2    3    4    5    6

30. I derive much strength from my
    relationship with God.                   1    2    3    4    5    6

31. My life is very fulfilled spiritually.   1    2    3    4    5    6

32. All my burdens have been lifted.         1    2    3    4    5    6

33. I started praying to God to deal
    with my problems.                        1    2    3    4    5    6

34. God's path is a joy of my life.          1    2    3    4    5    6

35. My interest in spiritual matters
    is increasing.                           1    2    3    4    5    6

36. I begin each day knowing that
    I am protected by the Higher
    Power.                                   1    2    3    4    5    6

37. I read spiritual writings daily and
    attempt to live my life accordingly.     1    2    3    4    5    6

38. I am trying to live my life accord-
    ing to the scriptures or according
    to moral principles of my beliefs.       1    2    3    4    5    6

39. I derive inner strength from my
    belief in a Higher Power.                1    2    3    4    5    6

40. Recently, spiritual matters have
    become more important to me
    than ever.                               1    2    3    4    5    6

41. I observe a special time for prayer.     1    2    3    4    5    6

42. My interest in spirituality has
    been revived.                            1    2    3    4    5    6

43. I have returned to some previous
    behaviors that I know are hurting
    me spiritually.                          1    2    3    4    5    6

44. I have fallen off a positive path
    that is important to me.           1   2   3   4   5   6

45. I have a renewed interest in
    spirituality.                      1   2   3   4   5   6

46. I have changed my behavior as a
    result of my spirituality.         1   2   3   4   5   6

47. I've lost my desire for spirituality.   1   2   3   4   5   6

48. I am straying away from my
    spiritual life.                    1   2   3   4   5   6

49. I am going through spiritual
    awakening.                         1   2   3   4   5   6

50. I believe that life is a great gift
    from God.                          1   2   3   4   5   6

## APPENDIX B

**Directions:** How would you describe yourself?

A. A spiritual person
B. A person with little or no interest in spiritual matters

If you consider yourself a spiritual person or a person with strong interests in spirituality, please answer questions under part A. If not, please answer questions under part B. Please limit your answers to two to three paragraphs.

### Part A: A Person with Spiritual Interests

1. Is spirituality important to you and why?
2. What are some of your spiritual beliefs?
3. How do you practice or put spirituality in your daily life?
4. When did you start taking interest in spirituality deliberately?
5. What specific incident/s do you recall which turned your life around to make you a spiritual person?
6. How would you describe your relationship with God or the Higher-Self?
7. To whom do you turn for help and hope when you are in deep trouble?
8. Who is your ultimate source of power? Who would you call upon for strength or special help?
9. How are your spiritual or religious beliefs helpful to you?
10. What is the most meaningful or important thing in your life?
11. Was there any major life event or trauma in your life which led you to become increasingly more interested in spirituality?
12. After changing path to spirituality, are there any behaviors that you had to curtail, shun, or stop?
13. After loss of interest in spiritual matters for some time, I am coming back with greater enthusiasm by engaging in many new behaviors such as:

14. I live my life in accordance with religious or spiritual laws. For instance,
15. I feel that I am in sync with the Higher Being, which makes me feel . . .

## B. A Person with Little or No Interest in Spiritual Matters

1. Why are you not interested in spirituality?
2. Could you share those incidents in your life that turned you off from spirituality?
3. Who would you turn to for help and hope when you are in deep trouble?
4. Who is your ultimate source of power? Who would you call upon for strength or special help?
5. What is the most meaningful or important thing in your life?
6. What are some of your beliefs about spirituality?
7. What made you interested in spirituality?

*(The author is grateful to Ms. Carolyn Sisk for sharing her spiritual autobiography with the readers. Thanks are also due to Scott Berry for his assistance).*

✍

# CHAPTER FIVE

# Weaving Sacred Threads into Multicultural Counseling

### Mary A. Fukuyama

I n the movie *Groundhog Day,* the main character lives the same day over again and again before he finally gets it right. Similarly, as I write this chapter, I experience déjà vu; that is, I repeatedly approach this expansive and ambitious topic with the hope that I refine it with each rendition, much like polishing a gemstone. I appreciate the structure and guidance offered by the editor of this unique, hands-on book. Accordingly, I will discuss the following topics: (1) my understanding of the relationship between spirituality and counseling, (2) the development of my personal interest in this topic, (3) spiritual perspectives in a case study, and (4) a summary and recommendations for training. It is my hope that this chapter will be an inspiration for engaging in spirituality and religion in counseling from a multicultural perspective.

## The Relationship Between Spirituality and Counseling

I see spirituality, religion, and culture as closely related, like the weaving of a tapestry—a heavy cloth with decorative designs and pictures woven into it. The fabric is made by interlacing threads or yarn on a loom. The warp, or vertical threads, runs lengthwise, providing the foundation for the fabric. The weft, or horizontal threads, adds different colors and creates the unique design.

Symbolically, the warp represents the depth and height dimensions or the essences of spirituality, for example, God or higher power, deepest level of meaning, and universal qualities of religion. The weft represents culturally diverse, religious, and individual expressions. The warp cannot exist without the weft; together they make a whole picture, a tapestry of unique design.

## Spirituality and Religion

What is meant by spirituality? Some definitions include descriptions like "the animating force in life, represented by such images as breath, wind, vigor and courage . . . an innate capacity and tendency to move towards knowledge, love, meaning, hope, transcendence, connectedness and compassion" ("Summit results," 1995). Other definitions focus on relationship: "a commitment to choose, as the primary context for understanding and acting, one's relatedness with all that is" (Griffith & Griffith, 2002, p. 15). Cornett offers yet another important dimension, that of mystery, "Spirituality is . . . the very essence of a view of the mysteries of life and, as such, a source of confusion, consternation, and conflict" (1998, p. 3).

How do these definitions of spirituality compare to definitions of religion? They are more alike than different. Paul Tillich described religion as the depth dimension of human existence. "Religion is the aspect of depth in the totality of human spirit . . . religious aspects point to that which is ultimate, infinite, unconscious in man's [sic] spiritual life. Religion, in the largest and most basic sense of the word, is ultimate concern" (1964, p. 7). The terms *religion* and *spirituality* are often used interchangeably, each with its own nuance. Artress (1995) has suggested that religion is like a container, such as a vase or cup, and spirituality— the essences held within. Returning to the metaphor of the tapestry, I view spirituality and religion as intimately intertwined.

## Culture

Both spirituality and religion must be understood in the context of culture. Again, many definitions of culture are in the literature, but I like this simple statement: "culture is comprised of patterns of beliefs, behaviors, and values that are maintained by a group of interacting people" (Bennett, 1996). It is an invisible web of meaning that is associated with nations, regions, ethnicity, and the workplace, as examples. Experts on cross-cultural communication highlight two types of culture: objective culture (institutions, systems, artifacts, customs, knowledge, etc.) and subjective culture (values, assumptions, and patterns of thinking). Subjective culture is associated with unconscious interpersonal processes, including communication styles (such as nonverbal communication), perception, language, and relationship dynamics (Stewart & Bennett, 1991).

Religion, as an institution and system, is imbedded in objective culture (such as houses of worship, doctrine, rituals, history), and it influences subjective culture, for instance, the individual's perceptions and worldview. Religion is both culture-specific and transcultural, that is, it goes beyond national boundaries. Finally, multiculturalism, by definition, recognizes that multiple realities co-exist; that is, many cultures, worldviews, languages, values systems, and customs serve to form diverse human communities (Sue & Sue, 2002).

Thus, I see multicultural counseling as primarily subjective and implicitly spiritual.

## Counseling

From a values perspective, counseling involves qualities of caring that are found in most religious and spiritual traditions: love, compassion, authenticity, and respect. Service, altruism, helping people, confrontation, challenge ("tough love"), and meaning- making are also spiritual dimensions for human growth and change. Some of these spiritual values will be discussed in the case study, particularly in "making meaning of suffering."

In addition, Carl Rogers's core therapeutic conditions, "congruence, unconditional positive regard, empathy, and a state of transcendence" have their roots in his theological training and religious background (see Murdock, 2004, pp. 125–127). Spiritual language has been incorporated into addiction recovery programs. Recent movements within counseling and psychology suggest that counselors address social justice issues, yet another spiritually rooted concern (Vera & Speight, 2003).

Most importantly, I consider the counseling relationship *per se* to have spiritual essences. Cornett has conceptualized Rogerian core conditions in psychodynamic language with the following emphases for the spiritually attuned therapist: "curiosity, a comfort with mystery, containment, empathy, amplification, and the willingness to look at one's own internal world" (1998, p. 140). Similarly, Griffith and Griffith emphasize fostering "curiosity, openness, and wonder as our dominant emotions in the therapy room" (2002, p. 48).

Experientially, when the counselor is "present" and in the moment in the therapy session, it invokes the numinous, similar to practicing the "I-Thou relationship," based on the works of twentieth-century philosopher Martin Buber (see Korb, 1988). To be truly present in the counseling session is a spiritual practice. Being aware of the "present moment" is a focus of mindfulness meditation (a Vipassana Buddhist practice) and contemplative prayer. Being in the moment has been explicitly incorporated into some therapy interventions, such as Gestalt therapy (Korb, 1988) or "focusing" (Gendlin, 1998). Cultivating present moment awareness is an engagement of attention that draws from transpersonal, creative, and spontaneous sources (Cortright, 1997).

Following trends from the feminist movement and postmodernism, spirituality is now being rediscovered (or uncovered, or revealed, or reclaimed) much as other disempowered voices have been restored to the therapeutic dialogue. Counseling as a profession is concerned with illuminating the soul (Cornett, 1998); even the word *psychology* is derived from Greek: *psyche* (soul) and *logos* (word).

Historically speaking, religion and psychotherapy have had an uneasy relationship. With the exception of Carl Jung, consideration of spirituality in psychotherapy has been marginalized. In fact, Gerald May noted that "within a generation after Freud's work became known, psychotherapy was in many circles supplanting spiritual and moral guidance as the primary method of alleviating mental disorders. There ensued an age in which psychologists and psychiatrists were seen by many as a kind of 'new priesthood'" (1982, p. 2).

The emphasis upon rationalism or scientific positivism has dominated counseling training. The influence of science and the scientific method on the counseling field has limited the inclusion of spirituality, because it cannot be easily reduced and studied objectively. In fact, science is limited to the study of observable and measurable matter, and spirituality encompasses a range of phenomena that are not easily subject to observation or measurement (see Huston Smith, cited in Cousineau, 2003). This emphasis on the scientific method has detracted from other ways of knowing, such as intuition, holism, and subjective experience. The issue here is not with science *per se* but with scientism, the imposition of the scientific worldview as the only source of truth.

The leaders in the transpersonal psychology movement of the 1960s, however, sustained a connection to the spiritual dimension (Cortright, 1997; Lukoff, 1998). Thus, I see counseling as a profession with spiritual and religious roots and infused with spiritual values and experiences.

### Attending to Spiritual Themes in Counseling

Although I have built a case for more similarities than differences between spirituality and counseling, I continue to study how to articulate religious and spiritual themes in counseling directly with clients. I offer several areas of concern: the nature of the Sacred, the complexity of cultural diversity, and understanding power dynamics.

There is an emphasis in western psychology on scientism, on being "in control" and for things to make sense, with reliance on empirically validated therapies as just one example. This emphasis is not conducive to opening to spiritual concerns. The nature of the Sacred in therapy, the first area of concern, entails skills of attending to subtle and symbolic language as well as listening to explicit stories (Griffith & Griffith, 2002). Engaging in dialogue about spiritual matters is a delicate process, sometimes facilitated by use of metaphors (Griffith & Griffith, 2002) and dream work (Taylor, 1993). To illustrate this point, I quote from Celtic spirituality:

> The world of the soul is a secret and sacred world, and you can't shine in on that world a light that is aggressive or that is too bright. . . . But sometimes the intensity and hunger with which people chase or try to hunt down the spiritual means that they actually never arrived there. Because the soul was never meant to be seen completely with the brightness or with too much clarity. The soul is always more at home in a light which has a hospitality to shadow. . . . Now in modern life, we have a neon kind of consciousness and much of the spiritual world is now completely pervaded with the language of psychology, and too often the language of psychology has a neon kind of clarity to it that is not able to retrieve or open up the depth and density of the world of soul.    (O'Donohue, 1996)

Regarding the second area of concern, one cannot assume in a pluralistic society such as the United States that counselor and client share the same worldview, which includes spiritual and religious beliefs and experiences. In fact, recognizing the complexity of cultural diversity, it is probably safer to assume that they do not. Counselors are particularly sensitive about not imposing their values or beliefs onto clients. This naturally leads one to view religion through the lens of cultural diversity, or in other words, acknowledging "that there are always multiple, alternative stories" (Griffith & Griffith, 2002, p. 31). The increased cultural diversity in the United States underscores the necessity for multicultural training for all mental health providers.

Demographic trends through immigration have influenced the diversification of American religious life (Hoge, 1996). I see an interaction of cultural diversity and religion in American culture, also influenced by an emphasis on individualism. Some people now describe themselves as "spiritual but not religious," and others pursue spiritual development through a mixture of culturally diverse expressions, which may be a unique American phenomenon (Lesser, 1999). It may not be so unusual, for example, for someone to attend a Methodist church service on Sunday morning, practice yoga on Wednesday evening, attend a lecture on Mindfulness Meditation and Stress Reduction on Thursday night, and volunteer at the homeless shelter on Saturday.

Power and privilege, the third concern, are discussed in depth in "oppression-sensitive therapy" (Nazario, 1998). It is essential to understand power dynamics, since psychotherapy or counseling is contextualized by sociopolitical dimensions that affect attitudes, perceptions, and behaviors. The therapist strives to form a collaborative relationship with clients, to achieve empowerment. It is important to note the power that is attributed both to the therapist and also to spiritual or religious symbols. Working with power dimensions in therapy at a conscious level is necessary to achieve the goal of empowering the client.

Zinnbauer and Pargament (2000) proposed various ways in which counselors may approach religion in counseling and suggested that the most compatible counselor orientations are the "pluralist" or the "social constructionist" because these positions allow for greater breadth of understanding culturally diverse clients. If a counselor's attitudes related to religion (either "for," in an absolutist way, or "against," in anti-religious stance) are particularly rigid, such orientations will limit understanding of diverse clients' religious or spiritual concerns.

Again, my understanding is that counseling is implicitly spiritual work. I am respectful of differences in the expressions of spirituality, particularly as expressed through religion and other cultural phenomena. My commitment is to multiculturalism as a foundation for addressing spiritual and religious concerns. I have found that immersion in multiculturalism can be a spiritually engaging, challenging, and expanding experience. The values that underlie multicultural work, such as flexibility, humor, and openness to differences may be synergistic with spiritual values, such as nurturing compassion, love, and authenticity (see Fukuyama & Sevig, 1999, p. 75).

## The Development of My Personal Interest in This Topic

There have been two major influences that affect my interests in multiculturalism and spirituality, both from my family of origin: first, ethnicity and the effects of racism, and second, my father, who was a Protestant minister and chaplain.

As I was growing up, I frequently encountered the question, "what are you?" I was easily mistaken for a Latina or an American Indian. My family history can be described as "mixed." That is, my father's parents were immigrants from Japan at the turn of the twentieth century, and my mother's Anglo-American heritage can be traced back to the English settlement of the colonies (Virginia). Racism played a significant role in my parents' lives. My father and his immediate family were put into relocation camps during World War Two, and this had a significant impact on our family history (Weglyn, 1976; Wilson & Hosokawa, 1980). Additionally, my parents' interracial marriage was a microcosm of cultural differences and religious commitment. Growing up as a biracial child, I learned about the necessity of bridging different worldviews (Fukuyama, 1999). From an early age, I realized that there was more than one way of expressing the Divine.

What was it like being a preacher's kid ("P. K.")? I grew up living literally next door to the church. Hence, I am comfortable with "God-talk." I am familiar with religion and how it functions both personally and in community. I am aware of its limitations and strengths. However, my interest in spirituality *per se* increased after my fortieth birthday. Developmentally this was a period of midlife crisis, which happened concurrently with my father's death from cancer. My curiosity about the interface of religion, spirituality, and the counseling profession also peaked. Multicultural counseling and training seemed like a natural place to focus this inquiry. Over a decade's collaboration with colleague Todd Sevig resulted in our publishing a book on the topic (Fukuyama & Sevig, 1999).

Now I would say that multiculturalism is normative for me. In addition to my family of origin, I am at ease with international travel and have been privileged to visit many countries around the world. I also identify as a global citizen (Fukuyama, 2003). My journeys have not all been easy, having experienced a difficult cultural immersion while volunteering in Guatemala, for example (Fukuyama, 2004). I have a healthy respect for the cultural adjustment process that is inherent with cultural relocation. All of these cross-cultural experiences have influenced my perspectives on religion; I see religion through the lens of cultural diversity. In addition, my awareness of multicultural dynamics has increased substantially, both at home as well as internationally.

I find that personal and professional growth in multiculturalism is inevitable and essential. There are two processes that provide the impetus and incentive to grow: (1) to ask good questions; in the words of Elie Wiesel, "There are no answers to true questions. There are only good questions" (1974, p. 276); and (2) to attend to feelings of discomfort.

In multicultural work, I find that it is necessary to move out of one's comfort zone in order to grow. On many occasions, my discomfort and resistance to the unfamiliar have been incentives to change and expand my consciousness and awareness.

It is safe to say that both my professional and personal life have been influenced by a wide variety of cultural and spiritual resources. My roots are in a Judeo-Christian heritage, and I continue to be an active member of an inclusive Christian church affiliated with the United Church of Christ, which has Congregational roots. However, as a lesbian and a woman, I am acutely aware of how religion can be unhealthy. This, too, has influenced my spiritual journey. Over the years, I have explored various religious paths including old-fashioned spiritism, pagan and sacred earth practices, women's spirituality (Christ & Plaskow, 1992; Flinders, 1998), contemplative prayer (May, 1982), Buddhist meditation (see writings by Thich Nhat Hanh, 1992), a Western form of Sufism (Fadiman & Frager, 1997; see works by Hazrat Inayat Khan, 1996) and Dances of Universal Peace (see *www.dancesofuniversalpeace.org/*).

I work at a publicly funded state university, primarily counseling with university students, teaching graduate-level courses, and supervising counseling trainees. I continually monitor the boundary between the secular and sacred, being respectful of separation of church and state, particularly in my teaching role. What this means is that I am careful not to impose a spiritual or religious view, and I seek to create safety so that all may express their spiritual views, whether in therapy or in the classroom.

I am fortunate to have colleagues at the University of Florida with whom I share the desire to weave spirituality into our work through teaching, research initiatives, and service to the community. The newly formed Center for Spirituality and Health (see *www.spiritualityandhealth.ufl.edu*) has sponsored course development, such as the one I teach on "spiritual issues in multicultural counseling," and other initiatives that bring together an interdisciplinary group of faculty, students, and interested community members. Together, we explore the interface of religion and science, spirit in the workplace and academic inquiry, and holistic perspectives in health care.

The Center also sponsors research initiatives, and I have enjoyed working with graduate students in a qualitative study on "multicultural expressions of spirituality," using focus groups and grounded theory. The Center has also sponsored research forums on spirituality in order to be better prepared to do research that incorporates this topic.

Because this is a fairly new area of discourse in counseling, I find the most rewarding experiences are in the classroom with colleagues, in our course Spirituality and Health, and in conversations with graduate students, as will be demonstrated in the case study. The benefits include finding deeper meaning in work and relationships, nurturing creativity, giving voice to important human process, and experiencing freedom from being professionally compartmentalized.

However, this work is challenging. It is difficult at times to hold a space for differences. In multiculturalism, cultural values are considered to be relative, that is, depending upon context, certain values may have more emphasis than others (for instance, individualism over collectivism). Religious values, however, tend to be "moral" and "absolute" by definition, with specific injunctions about what is right and wrong. Generally, people react to value differences, and prefer to think that their way is the right way. In a recent multicultural counseling course, one of the challenges for coming together as a group was religious differences, which included conservative Christian, atheist, antireligious, and universal points of view.

In addition to value differences, I am sensitive about crossing a boundary of the sacred in a secular setting. As teacher and counselor I am aware of the power in my role and make safety in the classroom a priority, a prerequisite for working together in the course. I am reluctant to engage in spiritual practices, even experimentally, in the classroom (if done, it is voluntary participation), but I encourage students to engage in spiritual practices outside of class.

In sum, I am happy to say that I am in good company in the growing body of literature and interests in spirituality and in multicultural counseling, with increasing numbers of conference programs and books being published on this topic (Burke & Miranti, 1995; Cashwell & Young, 2005; Frame, 2003; Kelly, 1995). It is complex to work in counseling with clients whose spiritual or religious beliefs are dissonant with how they see themselves. How do I know when religious or spiritual expressions are healthy or not? What is my role related to their spiritual beliefs? Do I challenge their beliefs? How relevant is counselor self-disclosure? These are some of the questions addressed in the case study that follows.

## Spiritual Perspectives in a Case Study

One way to clarify whether one's beliefs and practices are leading toward health and wholeness is through a process of discernment; that is, recognizing the fruits of one's actions. Are there positive or negative results? This issue will be addressed through selected passages from a verbatim transcript of a conversation with a graduate student on the meaning of suffering.

In this case, the student, who will be referred to by the initial "B" (details changed to protect confidentiality) is a fifty-year-old, white, female graduate student in the health professions. About a year ago, her father was severely burned. Within six months of his accident, her mother was diagnosed and died of cancer. Currently, her father has recovered from his injuries (he was near death) and returned to work. However, B has been depressed, questions her faith, and struggles to make meaning of suffering. She self-identifies as Buddhist.

B has expressed concerns about being angry all of the time, and is struggling with the question "why did this happen?" Buddhist practices helped her to cope with her father's injuries and recovery, but when her mother died, she started to question her beliefs. It seems that she is in a grief process related to her mother's untimely death and also experiencing a spiritual crisis. There are elements of both positive and negative expressions of spirituality in this case example. I refer to my responses by the letter "M." Brief commentaries are provided in italics.

*B:* Right . . . and so now I'm in the middle of just questioning what is. I wasn't the only one who went through that, my dad, my brother, and everything. My brother's faith is very strong; he is a fundamentalist Christian, and he's evidently able to weather this, or at least he is not telling me about his spiritual doubts, and he doesn't do much pondering over the nature of suffering. He just says, "Turn it over to God" or "let God handle it," but I am an analytical person, and I just want to know what's the point and what am I supposed to learn from all of this. Is there some sort of lesson, some karmic debt I need to work through, is there . . . (pause) if so, I'm not doing a very great job! [laugh]

*M:* Why do you say that?

*B:* Because I'm just angry all of the time! [laughter]

*M:* Oh, think you're not being grateful? [laughter]

*B:* Well, really . . . I have my moments of just outright hostility and that's . . .

*M:* About your mother's death?

*B:* About my mother's death and about my so-called friend, who more or less when things got really rough with my depression washed her hands of me.

*M:* hmmmm

*B:* And who now when I talk to her she acts like nothing happened, yet she never returns my calls or pages or anything, and we were really close, . . . and anger at my dad for getting burned. Anger just over lots of things and . . .

*M:* I understand anger to be an appropriate reaction to loss, but your anger is more than enough . . . for this loss and others? Or are you troubled by the amount of anger?

*B:* Yes, and I don't feel like I am being a good Buddhist actually, because I think anger is . . . you have to get really attached to something to get angry, and as Buddhist, one of the goals is to let go of attachment to worldly goods and your ego and negative emotions like anger and all of those sorts of things, so therein lies the spiritual crisis, I guess.

*Making meaning of suffering is one of life's greatest tasks. Religious beliefs such as "it's my karma" or "it's to teach me a lesson" may provide relief to some, but may negatively impact others. Sometimes, it is easier to "make meaning" once one has passed through the grief that one feels with a major loss, such as the death of a parent. Anger is a difficult emotion also, and sometimes spiritual or religious injunctions about expressing it complicate the grief process. In this situation, B was feeling a great deal of pain over the death of her mother, which was compounded by the preexisting trauma of her father's burn accident. Her interpretation of Buddhist teachings (to be detached from anger) is making her feel worse, so one might say that she is experiencing a negative form of spirituality, or perhaps caught in a "spiritual by-pass," that is, using a spiritual belief to avoid an inevitable human emotional process (grief). In addition, feelings of shame about not being "good enough" complicate her making use of her beliefs and practices. This illustrates the importance of having a teacher and community where one can get support and interpretation of religious principles.*

*Religions often have injunctions against anger. Cornett discussed the importance of addressing both love and hate (resulting in ambivalence) in order to heal "narcissistic injury" (1998, p. 82). He cautions, "In the denial and avoidance of anger, hatred, and related feelings, one not only lessens the intimacy available with the self and other people, one lessens the intimacy available with one's god" (1998, p. 100).*

*Norman Fischer, a renowned Zen teacher from the San Francisco Bay area, observed that a common error with Western practitioners of Buddhism is to believe "that suffering is something to be avoided, prevented, escaped, bypassed"*

*(2002, p. xvi). However, he suggests that "through the very suffering and the admission of suffering, the letting go into suffering and the calling out from it, mercy and peace can come." (2002, p. xvi). (Norman Fischer himself is a study of multicultural spirituality: He was raised in the Jewish tradition, studied Zen as an adult, experienced a Catholic monastic practice of singing the Psalms, and was inspired to translate selected Psalms into poetry from a Zen perspective.)*

*Later in the conversation, B says that she gets comfort from her spiritual practices.*

**B:** So in my heart I know that the practices are spiritually comforting, in my heart I know that, but in my intellect, my mind . . .

**M:** Your mind wants to know something your heart already knows. [laughter]

**B:** Yes, exactly [laughter] my mind and heart aren't talking to one another much lately . . .

*If this had been a therapy session, this moment would have provided a natural segue into Gestalt process, beginning a dialogue between the head and heart. It also illustrates different ways of knowing, and the point that spiritual wisdom may be accessed in more nonverbal and symbolic ways when compared to traditional scientific inquiry. A poem by Rumi expresses this well:*

> *O heart, sit with someone*
> *Who knows the heart;*
> *Go under the tree*
> *which has fresh blossoms.*
> *—Cited in Fadiman &*
> *Frager, 1997, p. 102*

*In this final selection, we continue to talk about expressions of anger and Buddhist perspectives on it. I also offer some self-disclosure, with the hope of normalizing the challenges of applying Buddhist principles to human emotions. I do not present myself as an expert, but as a fellow-journeyer. From an empowerment perspective, I would hope to model the search for meaning in a co-collaborative way.*

**M:** There's some sort of counterintuitive pieces to this, though, because to not feel pain, you tighten to not feel it, but then the tightening itself becomes painful, and so it's sort of counterintuitive to open to pain, it's like "I don't want to feel it," but the tightening ultimately becomes part of the pain.

*B:* It does, the anger just . . .

*M:* Do you see your anger as expressions of pain?

*B:* Um, I think so or as a protective mechanism, but it drives people away, and it just makes things worse, but it's easy to get really attached to it and tied into it, so I'm working in this clinic, a lot of patients I see are angry and hostile and going through their own [inaudible] mainly to do with finding [inaudible] and things like that. There's really a lot of bad energy there at that clinic.

*M:* So you can kind of see it in your face, I mean, it's like mirrored at you, and then you say, "so what about my own anger and attachment to anger and how healthy is that?"

*B:* Yes, exactly, yeah . . . not *very,* as far as I can see.

*M:* Well, maybe the Thich Nhat Hanh (2002) book on anger will help, but the lecture I heard him talk about anger was to really acknowledge anger but not acting on it, it's like breathing in, breathing out anger, and acknowledge it and see what happens, rather than "try not be angry," or the words get in my way [inaudible . . . laughter] which is . . . when I first heard him talk about it . . . I didn't get it, don't act on it, don't suppress it, so what are you going to do with it? Because . . . meditative practices are breathing in, breathing out . . . and just sitting with it.

*B:* And that's uncomfortable

*M:* He calls it cooking potatoes.

*B:* Oh no!

*M:* Cause he sees anger as like raw potatoes [editorial note: indigestible], and so you cook them and see what you get [editorial note: something nourishing].
The sitting with anger is cooking it.

*One other issue I think about is the question of "what authority do I have to speak about (insert any particular religious tradition)?" Are reading books, attending workshops, and periodically practicing meditations sufficient to offer spiritual guidance or interpretations? When is it appropriate to refer to specialists such as ministers, spiritual teachers, or a guru? Generally I am comfortable with referrals, and often I try to offer some spiritual suggestions, which I hope serve a positive psychological aim. However, I think this is an issue that merits ongoing consideration.*

## Concluding Thoughts

Integrating spiritual interventions in multicultural counseling is a complex matter. Considerations of counselor self-disclosure, dealing with value differences, and having knowledge of spiritual traditions are just a few of the issues. Bullis (1996) identified spiritual interventions used frequently by clinical social workers, which included recommending spiritual books, referral to spiritual leaders and/or community, exploring clients' religious/spiritual backgrounds, praying privately for clients, using religious/spiritual language or metaphors, and exploring spiritual elements in dreams. Generally speaking, I am comfortable with these kinds of interventions, but overall my concern is for client empowerment, and I enter into discussion of these topics with great tentativeness and respect.

Writing a chapter on spirituality and counseling such as this one was an opportunity for reflection upon themes that are core to my personal and professional life—exploring human nature at its best and weaving the sacred into my work as a multicultural teacher, trainer, and counselor. My own personal spiritual journey and multicultural background have given me insights into viewing religion and spirituality through a multicultural lens. As such, I am interested in exploring, that is, I am in search of that which is sacred and brings people into wholeness (the holy) in the context of multicultural counseling. As I engage in teaching and research on this topic, I am reminded that it is essential for me also to nurture myself in these dimensions (Palmer, 1997). I am grateful for this reminder.

In conclusion, I offer the following recommendations for training on the inclusion of spirituality and religion in multicultural counseling:

(1) Begin with self-awareness, understand the influence of family history, and resolve childhood issues and biases. I see some students entering psychology and counseling who have issues related to religion, and they still carry around old wounds, stereotypes, and negative images. I encourage individualized learning plans to move beyond these limitations.

(2) Learn about diverse religious and spiritual traditions, beliefs, and customs; increased exposure will reduce fears and misconceptions. Seek out personal experiences (beyond readings) through "action plans" (Parker, 1998). For example, visit worship services from traditions other than your own.

(3) Discuss topics with colleagues and in supervision. Cultivate safe places to have a conversation about religious beliefs and practices, and their intersection with mental health.

(4) Have a personal spiritual practice (walks in nature, centering breathing, church worship, yoga, tai-chi, etc.). I encourage students to select an activity of personal interest for starters, and for those who are experienced, I suggest that they select an activity that will deepen their "felt" spirituality.

(5) Study a spiritual tradition in depth for a period of time; "work it" before moving on. This is especially important for students who lack immersion in a spiritual tradition (see Lesser, 1999).

(6) Cultivate referral resources (minister, priest, rabbi, and spiritual director) who can serve as consultants.

(7) Talk with a trusted colleague with whom you can "check yourself" related to power issues or cultural blind spots. Spiritual work requires understanding the ego and its relationship to power.

(8) Be open to change. My experience is that the creative urges of the spirit require growth and change; for example, my spiritual perspectives and insights of ten years ago are no longer adequate for today, although they provide a good foundation.

(9) Enjoy the process!

Like a weaver, I am engaged in a co-creative process of discovering unique designs with spiritual, religious, and cultural dimensions. Hopefully with increased experience and awareness, the process of discovery will lead to appreciation of the beauty of unique tapestries, multicolored and textured.

## References

Artress, L. (1995). *Walking a sacred path: Rediscovering the labyrinth as a spiritual tool.* New York: Riverhead Books.

Bennett, M. (1996). Better together than apart, intercultural communication: An overview. Lecture presented to the Intercultural Communication Summer Institute. [Videotape available from Intercultural Resource Corporation, 78 Greylock Rd, Newtonville, MA 02160. Available online at *www.irc-international.com.*]

Bullis, R. K. (1996). *Spirituality in social work practice.* Washington, DC: Taylor & Francis.

Burke, M. T., & Miranti, J. G. (Eds.). (1995). *Counseling: The spiritual dimension.* Alexandria, VA: American Counseling Association.

Cashwell, C. S., & Young, J. S. (Eds.). (2005). *Spiritual and religious values in counseling: A guide to competent practice.* Alexandria, VA: American Counseling Association.

Christ, C. P., & Plaskow, J. (Eds.). (1992). *Womenspirit rising: A feminist reader in religion.* New York: Harper Collins.

Cornett, C. (1998). *The soul of psychotherapy: Recapturing the spiritual dimension in the therapeutic encounter.* New York: The Free Press.

Cortright, B. (1997). *Psychotherapy and spirit: Theory and practice in transpersonal psychotherapy.* Albany: State University of New York Press.

Cousineau, P. (2003). *The way things are: Conversations with Huston Smith on the spiritual life.* Berkeley: University of California Press.

Fadiman, J., & Frager, R. (1997). *Essential Sufism.* New York: Harper Collins.

Fischer, N. (2002). *Opening to you: Zen-inspired translations of the Psalms.* New York: Penguin Compass.

Flinders, C. L. (1998). *At the root of this longing: Reconciling a spiritual hunger and a feminist thirst.* New York: Harper Collins.

Frame, M. W. (2003). *Integrating religion and spirituality into counseling: A comprehensive approach.* Pacific Grove, CA: Brooks/Cole

Fukuyama, M. A. (2004). El Otro Lado. In E. A. Delgado-Romero & G. S. Howard (Eds.), *When things begin to go bad: Narrative explorations of difficult issues.* Lanham, MD: Hamilton Books.

Fukuyama, M. (2003). Spiritual responses to terrorism: Unity in diversity. In G. Roysircar, P. Arredondo, J. Fuertes, J. Ponterotto, & R. Toporek (Eds.), *Multicultural counseling competencies 2003: Association for Multicultural Counseling and Development* (pp. 61–68). Alexandria, VA: American Counseling Association.

Fukuyama, M. (1999). Personal narrative: Growing up biracial. *Journal of Counseling and Development, 77,* 12–14.

Fukuyama, M. A., & Sevig, T. D. (1999). *Integrating spirituality into multicultural counseling.* Thousand Oaks, CA: Sage.

Gendlin, E. T. (1998). *Focusing-oriented psychotherapy: A manual of the experiential method.* New York: Guilford Press.

Griffith, J. L., & Griffith, M. E. (2002). *Encountering the sacred in psychotherapy: How to talk with people about their spiritual lives.* New York: Guilford Press.

Hoge, D. R. (1996). Religion in America: The demographics of belief and affiliation. In E. P. Shafranske (Ed.), *Religion and the clinical practice of psychology* (pp. 21–41). Washington, DC: American Psychological Association.

Kelly, E. W., Jr. (1995). *Spirituality and religion in counseling and psychotherapy: Diversity in theory and practice.* Alexandria, VA: American Counseling Association.

Khan, H. I. (1996). *Sufi teachings: The smiling forehead.* London: East-West Publishing.

Korb, M. (1988). The numinous ground: I-Thou in gestalt work. *Gestalt Journal, 11*(1), 97–106.

Lesser, E. (1999). *The seeker's guide: Making your life a spiritual adventure.* New York: Villard.

Lukoff, D. (1998). From spiritual emergency to spiritual problem: The transpersonal roots of the new DSM-IV category. *Journal of Humanistic Psychology, 38*(2), 21–50.

May, G. (1982). *Care of mind, care of spirit: Psychiatric dimensions of spiritual direction.* New York: Harper Collins.

Murdock, N. L. (2004). *Theories of counseling and psychotherapy: A case approach.* Upper Saddle River, NJ: Pearson.

Nazario, A. (1998). Counseling Latina/o families. In W. M. Parker, *Consciousness-raising: A primer for multicultural counseling* (2nd ed., pp. 205–222). Springfield, IL: Charles C. Thomas.

O'Donohue, J. (1996) *Anam cara: Wisdom from the Celtic world,* Tape 1 "Your solitude is luminous." Audiotapes produced by Sounds True Audio, 735 Walnut, Boulder CO 80302. ISBN 1-56455-376-0. Order F039 800-333-9185.

Palmer, P. (1997). *The courage to teach: Exploring the inner landscape of a teacher's life.* San Francisco: Jossey-Bass.

Parker, W. M. (1998). *Consciousness-raising: A primer for multicultural counseling* (2nd ed.). Springfield, IL: Charles C. Thomas.

Stewart, E. C., & Bennett, M. J. (1991). *American cultural patterns: A cross-cultural perspective* (rev. ed.). Yarmouth, ME: Intercultural Press.

Sue, D. W., & Sue, D. (2002). *Counseling the culturally diverse: Theory and practice* (4th ed.). New York: John Wiley & Sons.

Summit results in formation of spirituality competencies. (December, 1995). *Counseling Today* (p. 30).

Taylor, J. (1993). *Where people fly and water runs uphill: Using dreams to tap the wisdom of the unconscious.* New York: Warner Books.

Thich, Nhat Hanh. (2002). *Anger: Wisdom for cooling the flames.* New York: Riverhead Books.

Thich, Nhat Hanh. (1992). *Peace is every step: The path of mindfulness in everyday life.* New York: Bantam.

Tillich, P. (1964). *Theology of culture.* New York: Oxford University Press.

Vera, E. M., & Speight, S. L. (2003). Multicultural competence, social justice, and counseling psychology: Expanding our roles. *Counseling Psychologist, 31,* 253–272.

Weglyn, M. (1976). *Years of infamy: The untold story of America's concentration camps.* New York: William Morrow.

Wiesel, E. (1974). Whatever I have learned in my life is questions. In A. Chapman (Ed.), *Jewish-American literature: An anthology* (pp. 276–278). New York: Mentor New American Library.

Wilson, R. A., & Hosokawa, B. (1980). *East to America: A history of the Japanese in the United States.* New York: William Morrow.

Zinnbauer, B. J., & Pargament, K. I. (2000). Working with the sacred: Four approaches to religious and spiritual issues in counseling. *Journal of Counseling and Development, 78,* 162–171.

❧

# CHAPTER SIX

# Breath of Heaven

## Craig S. Cashwell

> May all beings everywhere, with whom we are inseparably inter-
> connected, be fulfilled, awakened, and free. May there be peace in
> this world and throughout the entire universe, and may we all
> together complete the spiritual journey.
>
> —Lama Surya Das

Gratitude. This is the beginning place for me in writing this chapter. Gratitude to Oliver Morgan for undertaking such a work, and
gratitude for being invited to make a contribution to this book.

We know that the majority of persons in the United States consider
themselves to be religious or spiritual persons. Researchers suggest that
96 percent of persons living in the United States believe in God, over 90
percent pray, 69 percent are church members, and 43 percent have attended church, synagogue, or temple within the past seven days (Princeton Religion Research Center, 2000). Further, this does not begin to
count those persons for whom the primary expression of their spirituality
occurs outside of the context of organized religion. Eastern spiritual practices such as vipassana meditation, yoga, Reiki, tai chi, and qi continue
to increase in popularity in Western culture.

It follows, then, that many clients will come to us with openness and
a readiness to consider their spirituality as one aspect of their development and culture. In many cases, to ignore this aspect is to ignore a major
facet of the client's life. In fact, some models of wellness have suggested
that spiritual wellness is the core of overall wellness (Chandler, Holden &

Kolander, 1992; Myers, Sweeney & Witmer, 2000; Sweeney & Witmer, 1991; Witmer & Sweeney, 1992). It is my hope, then, that this book and, in a smaller sense, this chapter will contribute to the understanding of how spiritual practices that are consistent with client belief systems may be integrated into the counseling process to occasion spiritual experiences that facilitate client movement toward her or his Higher Self.

## Relationship Between Spirituality and Counseling

The relationship between spirituality and counseling remains fragile at best. Influenced by early writings, spirituality and counseling have often been considered as necessarily distinct. Freud characterized religion as *wishful thinking* and a *disavowal of reality* (Freud, 1927). Freud further suggested that the experiences of mystics were "infantile helplessness" and "regression to primary narcissism" (1930). Skinner (1945) character- ized religion as superstitious behavior perpetuated by an intermittent reinforcement schedule. Such negative evaluations are not relegated to the early and mid-part of the twentieth century, however. In a 2001 in- terview, Ellis stated that "spirit and soul is horseshit of the worst sort. Obviously there are no fairies, no Santa Clauses, no spirits. What there is, is human goals and purposes . . . a lot of transcendentalists are utter screwballs" (2001). Thus, some major theorists have characterized reli- gion and spirituality as pathological.

Other noted scholars and theorists, such as William James (1901) and Carl Jung (1970), however, have emphasized the central importance of religion and spirituality in the full development of a person. In more contemporary writings, scholars such as Assagioli (2000) and Wilber (2000) have also emphasized the centrality of religious and spiritual be- liefs and experiences.

How, then, have scholars arrived at such disparate conclusions about the role of religion and spirituality? I believe that one possibility is that they are all correct, at least to some extent. As an explanation, I use Wilber's (2000) template that religion and spirituality serve two pur- poses, one translative and one transformative. The *translative* purpose helps us make sense of a difficult world. For example, the Four Noble Truths of Buddhism teach that life is difficult because of our attach- ments. Religious and spiritual practices and experiences also serve a *transformative* purpose, enabling us to transcend our own ego-mind and connect to our Higher Self, a Self ordained to serve the highest common good, as in the further teaching of the Noble Truths, mentioned above, that the difficulty and these attachments can be transcended through living a compassionate life of virtue, wisdom, and meditation. Both purposes are essential.

Transformative experiences need integration. One example of a poorly integrated spirituality is the spiritual experience "junkie" who lives in near-constant need of the next spiritual high or fix. Such persons often ignore aspects of their day-to-day lives, such as work and social relationships, just as do persons with other addictions. Additionally, people who only experience the translative purpose of religion commonly reach a point where this is inadequate. Without transformation, their faith may falter.

Thus, it is in this context that we can understand how religion and spiritual practices can be either healing or destructive. A person who pursues religion for translation only, without pursuing personal growth, may become trapped in a position of emotional repression ("If you had enough faith, you wouldn't get angry"; "You shouldn't feel sad, he's in a better place") and extreme external locus of control that leads to abdication of personal responsibility for life ("Pray for healing instead of going to the doctor"). Ongoing experiences in religion solely for translative purposes may well lead to depressive symptoms or somatic complaints. Similarly, engaging in transformative spiritual practices without integrating (or translating) the experiences often leads to an undisciplined and unhealthy spiritual life; at an extreme, this can cause a breakdown rather than a breakthrough (Wilber, 2000).

For religion and spirituality to be healing, then, the translative and transformative purposes must be integrated. Unfortunately, I believe that we use the term *spirituality* rather loosely. "Are you a spiritual person?" we ask. This oversimplifies a complex interaction between beliefs, practices, and experiences. Ideally, there is a congruent flow between one's spiritual schemas (beliefs), behavior (practices), and the outcomes of these behaviors (experiences). In other cases, however, the three may not be so fluidly connected. One example of this is the aforementioned seeker of the peak experience who fails to work toward translating the experience or engaging in a disciplined spiritual practice to achieve a plateau state of being, considered by many to be more realistic and healthy than striving always for the peak experience. Another example would be the person who attends religious activities out of obligation ("I should go to church") without fully participating in the practices (such as prayer or communion) or opening to the experiences. Jung (1970) characterized such people as participating in religion to avoid having a religious experience.

There is a Hasidic tale that captures this point well:

> A Rabbi asked his disciples, "Where does God exist?"
> "God exists everywhere!", they cried with alacrity.
> "No," the Rabbi replied calmly. "God exists only where you allow God to exist."

For religion and spirituality to be healthy and appropriately integrated into the counseling process, then, I believe that several things must be true.

1. Any introduction of religion and spirituality into the counseling process must be consistent with the belief system of the client. This can only occur after a thorough assessment of client spirituality (see Harper & Gill, 2005).
2. The introduction of spirituality into the counseling process should include both the translative and transformative aspects.
3. Intention and attention should be applied toward a congruent flow between the client's religious beliefs, practices, and experiences. For many clients, this includes the introduction of disciplined spiritual practices that are consistent with their belief system.

## My Journey

There are many experiences, both positive and negative, that have influenced my interest in integrating spirituality into counseling practice. I will highlight some of these in this section. Before doing so, however, I want to emphasize that I believe that all counseling work is spiritual. The family-of-origin work that I did as a client twenty years ago and my experiences in Gestalt Groups over the past decade are as much a part of my spiritual history as my experiences in meditation groups, yoga classes, and Bible study groups. The spiritual path is, in my belief system, a path that leads inward toward the True Self or Higher Self. As such, the removal of any barriers along the path facilitates a more intimate connection with God. If at one point in a client's life, barriers are removed by deconstructing irrational beliefs, this is part of the spiritual path. At another point in the journey, a client may benefit most from emotional catharsis and integration. At another point, perhaps the changes a counselor helps the client make are behavioral. While the *content* of this work may not be explicitly spiritual, the *process* is nonetheless so.

Perhaps a brief case example is useful here. Lynn was a thirty-nine-year-old white female who presented for counseling with depressive symptoms. A very bright woman, Lynn reported that she had been through about two years of cognitive therapy with little symptom reduction, and wished to do experiential work. It became apparent through initial interviews that Lynn had great difficulty experiencing and expressing anger. It was equally apparent that she had a lot of anger that desired expression. Counseling afforded her the space to express her anger verbally, through dialogue experiments, and physically, through physical expression of anger within the session. Specifically, Lynn was encouraged to punch a pillow one day while she was expressing her anger. Though initially reserved in this action, she soon allowed the anger to flow more freely and fully expressed her anger both physically and verbally. I suppose there are some who would not consider a client screaming and flailing against a pillow to be spiritual work. Yet one outcome of our work together that Lynn reported is that her religious and spiritual life improved. She and I agreed that "emptying out" the anger created more space for the sacred in her life.

I suppose that my interest in religion began at birth. As the story is told, my mother was unable to take any medication for pain during my delivery and managed the pain by repeatedly reciting John 14:1–4 from the Christian Bible (May & Metzger, 1971):

> Let not your hearts be troubled, believe in God, believe also in me. In my Father's house are many rooms; if it were not so, would I have told you that I go to prepare a place for you? And when I go and prepare a place for you, I will come again and will take you to myself, that where I am you may be also. And you know the way where I am going.

Though the first sentence of this passage is a source of support for Christians, the full passage often is used during Christian funerals. How interesting, then, that it was a source of comfort to my mother during childbirth. In hindsight, this highlights for me the inextricable connection between birth and death.

I was blessed to grow up in a family where two distinct ways of thinking were modeled. My mother believed, or at least so it seemed to me, everything ever spoken by a minister from the pulpit. My father questioned, or again at least as it seemed to me, most of what ministers had to say. From this experience, I learned the place of faith, but also learned that the true path is one that is fraught with struggles and, ultimately, meaning that is highly personal. This would come to shape my experiences throughout my life.

Also, the church that I attended as a young child was rather evangelical, and the sermons seemed to focus on sin, unworthiness, and the very real possibility of eternal damnation. These experiences shaped my beliefs and practices as an adult as well. My personal belief system and life goal is to live from a place of love rather than fear. Yet, at the same time, I value the emotional passion that emerges within the spiritual path, whether this is a passion for a social cause or compassion for individuals met each day.

As an adolescent, I began to become disillusioned and bored with organized religion. In hindsight, I recognize that my religious activities were largely translative and that I was beginning to find this inadequate. I often saw and felt judgment within the church and was bothered by this. I also began to think about how a person's previous experiences affected how he or she viewed God and the role of religion. So, I suppose, began my interest in the interweaving of spirituality and counseling.

My disillusionment with organized religion found a point of focus in contemplative practice, or rather the lack of it, in the organized religion that I had experienced. I left the church during early adulthood for about seven years and began studying Buddhist meditation and other contemplative practices. These were my first experiences with world religions other than my own, and these experiences opened my eyes (and, perhaps, my heart) to the wisdom of traditions other than those with which I was raised. I was (and am) blessed with a life partner who understood this part of my journey, perhaps better than did I, and who supported my time away from organized religion while continuing to be involved in organized religion herself. Out of these experiences, I began to consider more fully issues of diversity in religious and spiritual beliefs and practices, and began to struggle with developing a disciplined spiritual practice that was my own.

The next transformative period began for me in my early thirties. My father was diagnosed with emphysema and relegated to oxygen, leaving him virtually homebound and clearly dying. As I struggled to come to grips with this, a close friend suggested that I go see a local woman (Jo) who performed a spiritual practice called Reiki (Japanese for *universal life energy*). I began to see Jo regularly, originally for what I thought would simply be stress management. Under her direction, guidance, and teaching, I began to have transpersonal experiences that opened me to a deeper communion with the Absolute. One benefit of this is that I became much more sensitive to the energy body and began to study and practice a range of energy-based practices, including chakra alignment (Pond, 1999), thought-field therapy (Callahan & Trubo, 2002), and breath therapy (Lampman, 1998; Taylor, 1994). I also was influenced by studies and practices within Native American traditions, such as shamanic journeying (Harner, 1990). So began a period of opening to the transformational aspects of spirituality.

During this period I also continued to study holy texts. One, in particular, the *Kabbalah,* stands out for me as important. The overarching learning for me from the *Kabbalah* was how essential it is to ground our spiritual practice. Stated another way, altered states are of no use unless they lead to altered traits (Smith, 2000). In exploring various spiritual practices and experiences, and in facilitating spiritual workshops and retreats, I have met many people whom I would characterize as ungrounded. These persons often had substantial problems with day-to-day functioning, such as maintaining intimate friendships and relationships and keeping a job. Such persons, I believe, have misused their spiritual practices to avoid psychological pain and unfinished business, a phenomenon referred to as *spiritual bypass* (Welwood, 2000). From this, I developed a personal commitment to grow and heal in all domains: the physical, emotional, cognitive, and spiritual. Further, my intention is that I remain firmly grounded while continuing my spiritual practice, and that I encourage this grounded approach to spirituality among clients.

A final thread that weaves throughout these developmental experiences is the importance of music. Singing in choral groups and listening to music from a variety of faith traditions has long been important to me. As my interest and knowledge of diverse spiritual traditions has grown, so too has my interest in diverse types of music. We are fortunate to live in a time when the music of many faith traditions can be so easily collected and enjoyed.

Now, as a middle-aged adult married for almost twenty years with a toddler daughter, I find myself humbled in hindsight at how these experiences together have shaped the importance of both the translative and transformative purposes of religion and spirituality in my life.

As might be expected, my interests in integrating spirituality into the counseling process have roughly paralleled my personal experiences. When my worldview of the purpose of religion was primarily translative (during my "antireligion" period), I saw no value in integrating spirituality into the counseling process and would not assess for spiritual and religious beliefs. If clients made statements about their faith, I would begin considering how their faith impeded their overall development. That is, I had a clear bias—a projection of my own experiences—

that active involvement in organized religion was not psychologically healthy. I can only pray now that the damage I did to clients in those years was minimal.

As I have grown to appreciate both the translational and transformational purposes of religion and spirituality, however, I have increasingly integrated spiritual assessment and intervention into my work. I now routinely include a variety of questions in early interviews with clients about their religious and spiritual history, beliefs, practices, and experiences. My intention is to assess without bias how religion and spirituality influence the presenting issue(s) of clients, and how spiritual practice may serve to complement or, in some instances, replace traditional talk therapy. I move now to discussing one particular case where spiritually oriented interventions became the primary focus of the counseling process.

## The Case of Sara

*Note:* Demographic information and some details have been modified to protect Sara's identity.

Because this case study involves the use of breathwork, I cite here the origin of some key words to transition to the case study. The root word for "spirit" is the Latin *spiritus,* which means "breath" or "breath of life." This was an attempt to translate the Greek noun *pneuma,* which means wind, breath, and life. Breath, and how breath connects us to spirit, is central to this case study. Finally, the words "healing," "whole," and "holy" all derive from the Old English *hal* and the Greek *holos,* suggesting that what is holy or spiritual is intimately connected to our health and wholeness.

Sara was a forty-five-year-old European-American female referred to me by another counselor. Sara had a history of depression and was taking antidepressant medication at the time of the referral. Sara had gone through a painful divorce twelve years previously that left her a single parent of two young children with very little financial or instrumental support from her ex-husband. She worked hard to provide for the family and even managed to earn advanced degrees over the next several years. This required her to overfunction in many different aspects of her life (financial provider, parent, student). She reported that her depression had gotten substantially worse as her second child prepared to leave for college, and that she began having some panic attacks at this time. Sara also had a long history of frequent and debilitating migraine headaches.

Doctors had prescribed several different medications, but none seemed to help substantially, and they often had numerous side effects.

Sara was referred to me by a counselor who was not interested in spiritually oriented approaches. The counselor reported that Sara was expressing frustration with the cognitive-behavioral work that they were doing together. She had said, "I've done all of this. This is not the answer. I want something different." Sara expressed a strong religious faith and a desire to work on the issues at a spiritual level. This occasioned the referral.

The first two sessions were largely spent exploring her history of depression and migraines, and her storied history of being in counseling, with most of this work being cognitive-behavioral in emphasis. Imbedded in this exploration, I asked her many questions about how religion and spiritual practice influenced these problems, such as:

- What do you value in life?
- What gives you a sense of purpose?
- How do you stay connected with your religion or spiritual path?
- How did marriage/divorce affect your religious or spiritual practices?
- What experiences have strengthened, diminished, or shaped your beliefs?
- How have your spiritual beliefs changed throughout your life?

I was cautious initially, using language in my questions that allowed Sara to discuss both positive and negative aspects of her religious and spiritual history, which she readily did. She spoke with a high level of awareness about the role that guilt played in her original family and her early religion, and how she had struggled to "dig out from under this mountain." She spoke, too, of the importance of prayer in her life. Further assessment indicated that her prayer life primarily included intercessory and petitionary prayer, and that she would pray during the migraines for the pain to be removed, which she believed helped the pain.

Sara was a quietly intense woman. She was extremely intelligent, having master's degrees in two fields and a Ph.D. She was very analytic and quick-minded. Late in the second session, I made a statement and asked a question that I commonly ask of students and clients like Sara. "You have a very sharp mind . . . and very sharp minds work quickly. That can be both a blessing and a challenge. How do you slow your mind?" Sara cast her gaze down and began to cry. She looked up and whispered, "I don't know." She went on to talk about her "quick mind" being a "thorn in my side." She reported problems sleeping because, as she said, "I can't turn it off. I worry that I may be doing something wrong at work, that I might not find another relationship, that the kids are okay, replaying a conversation from the workday, just whatever." Sara reported, "This wears me out. I'm tired all the time, but don't know how to turn it off."

Early in the next session, I asked Sara where she learned to think like that. Without hesitation, she said, "my mother . . . she's just like that." I suggested that there were possibilities for practices that would help with that, but that they would take time and disciplined practice, framing the problem of a "quick mind" as habituated learning that would take time to unlearn. This seemed to make sense to Sara and, I hope, created realistic expectations. We discussed various forms of meditation and types of prayer other than petitionary and intercessory.

The idea of contemplative prayer resonated with Sara, and we discussed the structure of this practice. She asked for a recommended reading on contemplative prayer. Knowing that her faith tradition was Christian, I recommended Keating's *Open Mind, Open Heart* (2000). As our relationship was clearly strengthening, I also playfully added, "You know, one possibility is that you might just start doing the practice without first analyzing it . . . that would be a different path for you." In hindsight, I believe that this was a divine moment in the counseling process where the "right thing to say" came through me rather than from me. I thought little of this statement, yet it was vitally important for Sara, as became apparent soon enough.

I expected that Sara would return the next week having read and reflected on *Open Mind, Open Heart* in its entirety. Such was her history of overfunctioning in all aspects of life. I was pleasantly surprised when a smiling Sara entered the next session saying, "I've got something that's going to surprise you." She went on to discuss how she had thought about my comment at the end of the previous session and decided to begin practicing contemplative prayer, using a spoken mantra, without first "analyzing it to death." She had practiced contemplative prayer for ten minutes a day for five days out of the previous week. This was the beginning of a transformative practice since her spiritual history had primarily involved translative study. This became an ongoing between-session assignment for her, one that she consistently followed; as might be expected, her capacity to quiet her mind improved.

From this, we began to discuss what our in-session work might look like. Sara said, "I think that contemplation is helping quiet my mind, and I plan to keep doing that. There's something more, though. I don't know what it is but I know it's not just talking about it." She went on to say that the most useful work she had done in the past had helped her express strong emotions. She had done some work with a Gestalt therapist and had participated in Radix Groupwork (Allison, 2001) to facilitate emotional expression. She stated, "I felt so alive when I did this work. My body, mind, and spirit all seemed on the same page. I didn't have migraines for weeks after that work, but then slowly they crept back in."

From the way Sara was talking about this, the mind-body connection and the potential for emotional release all seemed important. I introduced two possibilities for our work in session: Experiential Focusing (Gendlin, 1982) and Breathwork (Taylor, 1994). While the two approaches are technically quite different, the commonality between the two is that they bridge the conscious and the unconscious and help a person become more embodied, which seemed important for Sara. She responded that focusing sounded safer, then chuckled and said, "but since I'm in a mode of trying different things, let's try a breathwork session." After assessing for contraindications for breathwork, we scheduled a two-hour breathwork session for the following week.

## Breathwork

> The word BREATH implies more than the physical act of drawing air in and out of the lungs. Breath is the junction point between mind, body, and spirit. Every change of mental state is reflected first in the breath and then in the body.    (Deepak Chopra)

Breathwork involves a series of conscious connected breathing strategies to clear out physical, mental, and emotional blocks. The breathing processes used in breath therapy are the opposite of the types of breath holding used to repress these blocks; the conscious connected breathing strategies trigger a natural process of cleansing and purifying in both the body and the psyche (Lampman, 1998). Breath therapy serves the multiple purposes of promoting personal growth, stress management, spiritual development, and is a logical adjunct to counseling or psychotherapy (Lampman, 1998). There are a variety of similar but distinct approaches to breathwork, including holotropic breathwork (Grof, 1998), integrated breathwork (Manne, 2004), and breath therapy (Lampman, 1998). The approach with Sara described here is based on Lampman's breath therapy.

The initial breathwork session consisted of assessing her normal breathing pattern, teaching the primary breath patterns, setting an intention, and then facilitating the breath session. To set her intention, I

asked Sara to close her eyes, breathe into her heart, and allow her intention for the breath session to emerge from her wisdom rather than her
knowledge. Sara set an intention that surprised me somewhat. She said,
"My intention is to release the blocks that keep me from speaking my
mind." This was not a topic that we had processed at any length in previous sessions. In her initial session, Sara experienced a strong emotional
release of sadness about working too hard and thinking too much.

One issue with which I struggled internally with Sara was the extent
to which we should process the sessions. On the one hand, I knew that
the integrative aspect of the process was important. On the other hand,
I knew also of Sara's history of being overly analytical. My own experiences as a "breather" lead me to believe that many of the experiences
that occur in such a deep level of consciousness often defy logic from the
conscious ego mind. So, we processed briefly, mostly about how she was
feeling after the session ("terrific," she smiled). Sara said this was just
what she wanted and, with encouragement to continue her contemplative prayer practice, we scheduled another breath session.

Prior to the next session, Sara reported only one headache in the previous week and that it was nowhere near her usual migraine intensity.
In the second session, Sara set her intention: To release fear. I think that
Sara expected we would verbally process this before moving into the
breath session, but I had the intention to move away from the analytical talk approach and to move immediately into the breath session once
an intention was set. Though several things happened in this session,
one seems most noteworthy. At one point, Sara, touched her heart and
whispered, "It's getting cold." The intensity of her breathing changed,
and she moved her hands over her face and then over her head. A few
minutes later, Sara extended her arms and her fingers began twitching
as if reaching for something. As breath therapists are trained to do, I
gave her "grasping" hands something to grasp, in this instance my own
hands. She quickly grasped my hands, tugged on them gently, and held
on throughout the remainder of the session. Soon after this, Sara verbal-
ized that she could feel the energy pulsing up and down her body. She
quickly added, "it's not bad . . . it's good . . . REAL good."

She rested in this space for a few minutes and then said something that
was, I believe, a turning point for her work. She started laughing and said,
"It makes no damn sense . . . and that feels good." Her laughter increased,
and I spontaneously began a guttural laugh with her. After the session, I
reflected in my journal how ironic and wonderful that I was laughing hys-
terically with a client because she did NOT understand something.

In her third breath session, Sara set her intention to release undesirable emotions. She reported a situation where a co-worker wanted her to do work that was the responsibility of the co-worker. Sara had a very strong emotional reaction to this that she still felt in her body. As she began conscious connected breathing, she fairly quickly articulated, "It's not my job . . . why do you want me to do your work for you?" Soon after, she said, "I don't want to meet expectations . . . I can't . . . It's so far back about meeting somebody's expectations, trying to but being pissed, withdrawing, getting sad, getting afraid, choosing jobs that depend on me, what I have to do, not what other people do." She then stated, "It hurts" and pointed to her chest. "If I don't do it, something will happen . . . something bad." While many things happened in this session, the most noteworthy is that she connected three different experiences that occurred between her and her mother when she was age four, five, and twelve. The commonality in each of these experiences was that her mother held developmentally inappropriate expectations of her, and Sara felt both angry and sad about these occurrences. This is referred to as linked trauma or condensed experiences (Grof, 1998) and is common during breathwork sessions. From this session, Sara gained insight about the source of her painful experience earlier in the day, providing her some direction for self-healing.

Sara went on to have an additional eight breath sessions. There were many wonderful experiences, including emotional releases and, in later sessions, some wonderful transpersonal experiences in which Sara came into close communion with her Higher Power. Unlike the tears of release, in these sessions she cried tears of bliss and joy. One common occurrence across these sessions was that Sara would experience the physical sensations that she had when a migraine began, but without migraines. Throughout the experience, Sara began to bring a journal and spontaneously record her experiences at the conclusion of each session. As she moved further into her breath practice, we also began to use postsession Mandala drawings to help her integrate her experiences at the end of the session.

Once people complete ten to twelve breath sessions, they may reach a point where it is safe to do breath sessions without a sitter. I made the decision that this was the case for Sara, who increasingly needed less and less guidance and direction from me in each session. I encouraged Sara to continue her contemplative prayer practice (which by then was up to twenty minutes a day with fewer moments of distractedness) as the foundation of her work, and to do one or two breath sessions in the coming week. We treated this as a possible termination of our work together, with an open invitation to return if she felt she needed me to facilitate additional breath sessions, or if she had experiences that she believed she needed help integrating.

Sara called me about five weeks later, simply as an update. She reported that her contemplative prayer practice was continuing to strengthen and that she now recognized that she could quiet her mind at any point in her day by spending just a few moments in contemplative prayer. She also reported doing two breath sessions every week and that she was continuing to gain insights and release negative emotions that she had stored in her body. She also reported that she was spending less time at work and was beginning to volunteer her time at a children's hospital. I encouraged her to continue what she was doing and to contact me in the future if she needed additional assistance. As I was writing this chapter, Sara contacted me to let me know that she had used a breath session to gain clarity about a major life decision and that she was grateful for our work together. I, too, feel blessed by the privilege to work with Sara.

## A Caveat

Though Sara's experiences in breath work are not uncommon, there are many clients who will not benefit from this type of work. Most notably in my experience are those persons who are not open to alternative approaches to the therapeutic process and those unable to *surrender* to this process. If clients are open to the approach and willing to stay with the process and work through any resistances they may experience, however, breath therapy may provide a valuable experience.

I chose to include the case of Sara because I think it exemplifies the main themes I have tried to develop in this chapter. Sara's spiritual history had largely been translative, and I was fortunate to work with Sara at a point in her life at which she was yearning for more from her spiritual life. She longed for transformation. The combined practice of contemplative prayer and breath therapy helped Sara integrate her beliefs, practices, and experiences more fully in her everyday life.

## Concluding Thoughts

The integration of spirituality into counseling practice is a logical blend. It is unfortunate that some, in pathologizing religion and also confounding religion and spirituality, have refused to consider the healing and growth that are possible through spiritual practice and experiences, and the meaning-making that may emerge from spiritual study and development of an integrated belief system. I believe there are three issues to which I must consciously attend if I continue to integrate spirituality into my clinical practice. I offer these here as recommendations for those who want to more systematically attend to the spiritual in their counseling practice or training:

1. *I will do my own work.* Whatever form this takes, continue developing your own path. For me, this takes many forms, including daily meditation and yoga, participating in an experiential therapy group, breathwork sessions, and as much time as possible spent in nature.

2. *I will learn.* We are fortunate to live in a time when the wisdom of faith traditions and spiritual practices are readily available through various forms of media. Study and learn about diverse belief systems, spiritual practices, and spiritual experiences.

3. *I will participate in a community (or communities) that support my growth.* Whether this be a group founded around religious beliefs, or a community of spiritual practitioners (or both), it is important to engage in dialogue and practice with people of like mind. We grow through our relationships with other people.

In conclusion, the personal journey toward wholeness is one that incorporates spiritual beliefs, practices, and experiences such that life is more fulfilling, enriching, and complete. The same argument can be extended to my work as a counselor. If I perceive a client as solely a cluster of symptoms that need alleviation, reduction of these symptoms is the best that we can hope for in our work together. If, however, I perceive a client as pure consciousness that has been wounded over time, and strive to facilitate the client's holotropic development (that is, moving toward wholeness), both therapeutic process and outcomes are impacted in a way that serves a much higher good.

Note: For information on training in breath therapy, please see *www.breaththerapy.net.*

## References

Allison, N. (2001). *The complete body, mind, and spirit.* Columbus, OH: McGraw-Hill.

Assagioli, R. (2000). *Psychosynthesis: A collection of basic writings.* Amherst, MA: The Synthesis Center.

Callahan, R., & Trubo, R. (2002). *Tapping the healer within: Using thought-field therapy to instantly conquer your fears, anxieties, and emotional distress.* Columbus, OH: McGraw-Hill.

Chandler, Holden, J., & Kolander, C. (1992). Counseling for spiritual wellness: Theory and practice. *Journal of Counseling and Development, 71,* 168–175.

Ellis, A. (2001). An interview with Albert Ellis. Available at *www.psychotherapist resources.com/current/cgi/framemaker.cgi?mainframe=totm&subframe=ellis.*

Freud, S. (1927). *Future of an illusion.* New York: W. W. Norton.

Freud, S. (1930). *Civilization and its discontents.* New York. W. W. Norton.

Gendlin, E. (1982). *Focusing.* New York: Bantam.

Grof, S. (1998). *Adventures in self-discovery.* Albany: State University of New York Press.

Grof, S., & Grof, C. (1989). *Spiritual emergency: When personal transformation becomes a crisis.* Los Angeles: J. P. Tarcher.

Harner, M. (1990). *The way of the shaman.* San Francisco: Harper.

Harper, M., & Gill, C. (2005). Assessing spirituality. In C. S. Cashwell & J. S. Young (Eds.), *Spirituality in counseling: A guide to competent practice.* Alexandria, VA: American Counseling Association.

James, W. (1901). *The varieties of religious experience.* London: Collins.

Jung, C. G. (1970). *Collected works of C. G. Jung: East and west: Psychology and religion.* New York: Taylor and Francis.

Keating, T. (2000). *Open mind, open heart: The contemplative dimension of the Gospel.* London: Harper Collins.

Kurtz, E., & Ketcham, K. (1994). *The spirituality of imperfection: Storytelling and the search for meaning.* New York: Bantam.

Lampman, C. (1998). *Breath therapy training—Level I Manual.* Tucson, AZ: Integration Concepts.

Manne, J. (2004). *Conscious breathing: How shamanic breathwork can transform your life.* Berkeley: North Atlantic Books.

May, H. G., & Metzger, B. M. (1973). *The new Oxford annotated bible.* New York: Oxford University Press.

Myers, J. E., Sweeney, T. J., & Witmer, J. M. (2000). The wheel of wellness counseling for wellness: A holistic model for treatment planning. *Journal of Counseling and Development, 78,* 251–266.

Peers, E. A. (Translator and editor). (1990). *Dark night of the soul: A masterpiece in the literature and mysticism by St. John of the Cross.* New York: Image.

Pond, D. (1999). *Chakras for beginners: A guide to balancing our chakra energies.* St. Paul: Llewellyn.

Princeton Religion Research Center (2000). Americans remain very religious, but not necessarily in conventional ways. *Emerging Trends, 22*(1), 2–3.

Skinner, B. F. (1945). *Walden Two.* New York: Prentice Hall.

Smith, H. (2000). *Cleansing the doors of perception: The religious significance of entheogenic plants and chemicals.* Los Angeles: Jeremy Tarcher.

Sweeney, T. J., & Witmer, J. M. (1991). Beyond social interest: Striving for optimum health and wellness. *Individual Psychology: Journal of Adlerian Theory, Research, and Practice, 47,* 527–540.

Taylor, K. (1994). *The breathwork experience: Exploration and healing in non-ordinary consciousness.* Santa Cruz, CA: Hanford Mead.

Welwood, J. (2000). *Toward a psychology of awakening: Buddhism, psychotherapy, and the path of personal and spiritual transformation.* Boston: Shambhala.

Wilber, K. (2000, May). A spirituality that transforms. *Tools for transformation newsletter.* Available at *www.trans4mind.com/news/kenwilber.html.*

Witmer, J. M., & Sweeney, T. J. (1992). A holistic model for wellness and prevention over the life span. *Journal of Counseling and Development, 71,* 140–148.

# CHAPTER SEVEN

# Remembering the Lessons
# of the Angel

## Rebecca Powell Stanard

> Just before a baby is born, an angel shows it everything there is to
> know and learn on Earth. Then at the moment of birth, the angel
> touches the infant's nose, and the child forgets everything. We
> spend the rest of our lives remembering what the angel showed us.
> —Jewish teaching

This story delights me because it seems to be an accurate metaphor
for my life. I am a fully human, fifty-something-year-old female who
struggles with an ever-changing understanding of the world and my place
in it. I am a counselor-educator and a practicing counselor. For my ideal
self, spirituality is a way of being, a guiding force for how I live my life
and how I interact with others. It influences my professional life in the
way I work with my students and clients. My real self struggles to remember this on a moment-to-moment basis.

I have the sacred privilege of being with clients as they grapple with
the painful realities of their lives. I am also with them as they access
within themselves an understanding that transcends the pain and leads
them to discovery of meaning and purpose in their lives. That understanding is derived from their true nature, their spiritual nature. That
spiritual nature is our birthright. Our human experiences are deeply
painful at times, but they provide us with an opportunity to reconnect,
rediscover our true self, our spiritual nature, and to discover meaning,

purpose, and even joy. We are given the opportunity to remember what the angel taught us before we were born.

This spirit, this knowledge, this understanding, this power—what is it? What is its origin? How can one access it? The truth is, I don't always know, and I don't know universal answers, only personal ones. Those answers are ever changing as I discover new questions and have new experiences. So all I have to offer is my understanding at the present moment.

## A Personal Understanding of Spirituality

> In midwinter, Saint Francis called out to an almond tree "Speak to me of God." The almond tree burst into bloom. It came alive. (Christian legend)

Spirituality is the always available present-moment experience of a power that transcends the limitations of human intellect and ego. Its presence leads to a deep, genuine understanding and loving acceptance of one's authentic self. Its power connects us to one another and to all of creation. Spirituality is mysterious, powerful, life-affirming, and transformative.

What is the source of this power? Deepak Chopra (1995) says that we are spiritual beings that have taken manifestation in physical form. I believe our spiritual being is of God. It is not bestowed by the conceptual God, not the Christian God, the God of Islam, the Jewish God, nor any other God, but the living breath of God that transcends religious concepts. It may be called by many names: Holy Spirit, Higher Power, or Buddha nature; whatever the name ascribed to it, it is the spirit that dwells within each of us that is our authentic nature. Spirituality is our awareness of that reality.

> Chop wood. Carry water.    (Buddhist teaching)

Spirituality is always available to us. It is as near as our breath. But we can only experience it when we are mindful and present to life. Because it is an experience, words are inadequate to describe it. An experience described is one that is no longer present-moment but one whose moment has passed. How can I, today, possibly convey to anyone else the experience of cool water on my hands as I stood before a sink on a late summer afternoon long ago, washing the abundant harvest of dark purple concord grapes from my arbor? How can I describe the experience of the sun warming my kitchen, my skin, and my soul, the sweet smell of the grapes, the beauty and joy of the sound and sight of my children laughing and playing in the yard as I worked, or the sweet sound of music in the air? I can remember the clarity and power of that moment from years ago. I was connected to all life—past, present, and future. I knew who I was. I understood the meaning of my life at that moment. I was transformed. I can't fully recapture in words the experience or the meaning of that moment for myself much less convey it to anyone else. What was it about that particular moment that made it different from thousands of similar moments in my life?

I believe that it was different because I was different. I was fully present, and that presence allowed me to access the joy, power, and understanding that are always available to each of us when we are simply mindful. Spirituality may be the big moments deliberately sought after, but, in my experience, it is more often found in simple human acts done with presence and mindfulness.

> Always remember you are unique, just like everybody else.
> (Tom Everhart)

Spirituality is paradoxical. It is both personal and universal. My private and seemingly personal spiritual experiences are often universal when shared with another. There is an understanding of the shared meaning of our seeming disparate experiences. It is a touching of our spirits that transcends our intellectual understanding. In fact, the more I struggle to understand, the more understanding eludes me. It is only when I give up the struggle, when I give up knowing, that understanding comes. It is a profound understanding that takes place in moments of crystal clarity. It comes from deep within, often in quiet moments. It comes when I get out of my head and into my heart. As Carl Jung stated, "Your vision will become clear only when you can look into your own heart. Who looks outside, dreams; who looks inside, awakes" (Simpson, 1988).

> When I was a child, I spoke like a child, I thought like a child,
> I reasoned like a child; when I became a man, I gave up childish
> ways.    (1 Corinthians 13:11).

Spirituality is a developmental process. Fowler (1981) speaks of it in terms of faith development. While he uses the word *faith,* his definition of faith is more broadly defined than the traditional use of the word and is similar to definitions of spirituality. Fowler conceptualizes faith as a generic human phenomenon, a way of relating and knowing. It may or may not be traditionally religious. In his six-stage model, individuals move from blind acceptance of the beliefs and values of their religious communities, as taught to them by the significant adults in their lives, to more questioning and inclusive attitudes. It culminates in a universal spirituality that extends beyond any specific religious belief.

I've experienced this development as a process of growing into authenticity, a process of becoming, of growing into an awareness of my true nature. Spiritual development requires that I let go of my false self, my ego, in order to access my true self, my spiritual self. It requires a willingness to let go of the security of knowing for the insecurity of ambiguity. When I am unsure, when I don't have all the answers, when I am genuine, then I can connect with another human being. I've come to believe that the only authentic human encounters are spiritual encounters. All others are ego. It took me a long time to understand this. I still get scared and forget it.

> This is my simple religion. There is no need for temples; no need for complicated philosophy. Our own brain, our own heart is our temple; the philosophy is kindness.    (H.H. the Dalai Lama)

I know deeply spiritual people both within and outside the confines of religion. True spirituality transcends religious beliefs. The common element of spirituality among those who claim no religious affiliation and those of various faiths is awareness of a power greater than oneself that is part of the self. According to the Christian tradition, "All those who are led by the Spirit of God are sons of God" (Romans 8:14). The Dzogchen Buddhist master Lama Surya Das (1997, p. 15) says, "We are all lit up from within as if from a sacred source" and that we are all living Buddhas whose only task is to awaken to who and what we are. The Qur'an teaches that "He is with you, wherever you are" (57:4). While different faiths have different roots, traditions, and beliefs, a potential unifying factor is acknowledgment of our innate spiritual nature. That spiritual nature can be a powerful force for healing in the world. Thich Nhat Hanh quotes Professor Hans Küng, "Until there is peace between religions, there can be no peace in the world" (1995, p. 2).

Spirituality is a powerful transformative force that has been long neglected by the counseling profession. It is a force whose time has come. The professional literature is replete with articles that extol the benefits of incorporating spirituality into counseling. How does one go about that? Like all interventions, I think this approach requires that counselors have a personal understanding of the nature of counseling and of their own theoretical and spiritual orientation, so that counselors do not impose their own values on the client. It requires an openness, acceptance, and willingness to learn about various spiritual and religious traditions. It is exciting and fertile new ground for our profession.

## A Personal Understanding of Counseling

Life is difficult.    (The First Noble Truth in Buddhist tradition)

People seek counseling because life is painful and they are overwhelmed by the pain. Their pain and suffering is often simply the result of the human condition: sickness, disease, death, loss, abandonment. Sometimes, their pain is the result of difficulty accepting the fact that life is ever changing. They cling to the past or look longingly toward some idealized future. Other times, they seek counseling because their life is unsatisfying and they don't know why or what to do about it. They are trapped, living a life circumscribed by others. They don't know who they really are or how to become the person they want to be. They come seeking relief from their suffering. How can we effectively use the power of spirituality to help clients move beyond the suffering to live more authentic, satisfying lives?

The touchstone of validity is my own experience.    (Carl Rogers)

I am, by nature, existential; by training and experience, person-centered; and by spiritual orientation, Buddhist. I believe that there is meaning to life's experiences. I believe that within each of us is the desire to tap into that meaning and that, given the appropriate conditions, we have the ability to do so. I believe that by nature we are all Buddhas. My experiences personally, professionally, and spiritually have validated those beliefs.

My work as a counselor and as a counselor educator is shaped by my experience and those beliefs. I am profoundly influenced by the work of Carl Rogers. It is compatible with my beliefs and experiences. The central tenet of person-centered counseling is that individuals have within themselves the capacity for self-understanding and that, in a facilitative therapeutic relationship, they can effectively use those resources to alter their self-concept, attitudes, and behaviors (Rogers, 1980). The three conditions that Rogers identified as necessary for the establishment of this growth-producing relationship are genuineness, unconditional positive regard, and empathic understanding. The relationship is the key to unlocking the change process in the individual. The relationship allows for the emergence of true self.

I believe that person-centered counseling is not only compatible with spirituality, but is itself a spiritual intervention. It involves the creation of a space in which the client feels safe to reveal him- or her-self to another. I consider this space to be sacred because it is a place where two souls meet, a genuine relationship is formed, and the opportunity for wholeness is revealed. It is in this sacred space that clients feel free to just "be" and to explore the meaning of that "beingness." Rogers himself conceptualized the encounter that occurs in that space in spiritual terms. "It seems that my inner spirit has reached out and touched the inner spirit of the other" (Rogers, 1980, p. 129). I, like Rogers, value the touching of spirits as a sacred experience for both the client and myself. "Our experiences in therapy and in groups, it is clear, involve the transcendent, the indescribable, the spiritual. I am compelled to believe that I, like many others, have underestimated the importance of this mystical, spiritual dimension" (Rogers, 1980, p. 130).

I didn't always "know" these things, even though some of them were taught to me in graduate school. I learned from my experiences working with clients. I've grown into understanding as part of a developmental process that parallels my development personally and spiritually. When clients came to me in their pain, seeking help, I tried all the tools I'd acquired in my graduate training to help them. Sometimes, it was beneficial, but often the relief was temporary, and the process was ultimately unsatisfying for both of us. The more I tried to be an "expert," the less satisfying and successful the counseling outcomes were. I came to understand that often my client and I were trying to solve human problems with human solutions. Einstein (1956) said that a problem cannot be solved from the same level of consciousness that created it. The human problems that bring people into counseling often require a higher level, a higher way of knowing and understanding. I believe that higher level is the spiritual level and that person-centered counseling allows me to communicate with people on that level because it creates a safe place in which an authentic encounter can occur.

> The most precious gift we can offer others is our presence.     (Thich
> Nhat Hanh)

When I can be genuine, offer unconditional positive regard, and listen empathically, I am truly present in the relationship. I can do that only when I am stripped of ego and accessing my true nature, my spiritual nature.

My ability to do that leads to a genuine presence that facilitates a climate of acceptance in which the client experiences self-acceptance. Rogers (1961) says that change cannot occur without this self-acceptance. This self-acceptance frees the client to live his or her life more effectively. Our journey together becomes more about the questions than about the answers. The client begins to ask deeper questions like "Who am I?" and "How may I become myself?" These are deeply spiritual questions that require spiritual answers.

### Translating Understanding into Practice

I've found many different ways to work with clients to explore those spiritual questions. The work must be done in a way that honors the client's spiritual beliefs and traditions. I work in the South, the cradle of fundamentalist Christianity. Many, if not most, of my clients have spiritual traditions and beliefs vastly different from mine. I'm aware of that. They generally are not, because I work with them in the context of their values and beliefs. I am able to connect with them by operating at the level of our spiritual nature, whether one calls it Holy Spirit, Buddha nature, or some other name. The spiritual level transcends our religious differences. It allows us to explore the events of their lives and discern meaning from them. The connection facilitates growth and change. The following case discussion illustrates my integration of spirituality into the counseling process.

## Liz's Journey

Liz was a forty-year-old intelligent, articulate, white female who was referred by her psychiatrist for treatment of posttraumatic stress disorder (PTSD). She was suffering from intrusive dreams, flashbacks, difficulty sleeping, and anxiety attacks associated with an automobile accident that had occurred six months earlier in which the driver of the other automobile was killed. Liz presented with a great deal of anxiety about the counseling process itself and made it clear that she liked structure and needed to maintain control of our work together. She acknowledged that the accident and the symptoms of her PTSD were problematic for her, but they were related to things that were more frightening to her. "All of the stuff in unopened boxes that I've pushed to the side and I'm afraid to open." She made only oblique references to numerous unresolved issues that she wanted to explore but of which she was afraid. I honored her fear and offered her reassurance that we would "open the boxes" and explore them only if and when she indicated she was willing and able to do so.

Liz was confined to a wheelchair as a result of a progressive neurological disorder that she had been diagnosed with as a child. The diagnosis of that disorder was problematic, and in addition to suffering from vague symptoms, numerous hospitalizations, trauma, and pain, she also felt neglected by her parents, particularly her mother, who believed that Liz was malingering. Liz described numerous dissociative episodes during her childhood, again only indirectly alluding to the traumatic events that precipitated them. The automobile accident had triggered a fear in her that she could no longer control these episodes and that indeed her life itself was spinning out of control.

Liz worked as a technical writer for a large company. She also liked to write short stories and paint. We agreed in our first session that she could use her interest in writing to keep a dream journal so that we might explore her vivid dreams. We also talked about expressing herself through her artwork. She informed me that she had been in the process of painting a picture of a black bear but had been unable to finish it. It somehow was linked to the unfinished areas of her life, and she would finish her picture when she finished her work in counseling.

Spirituality was introduced early in the counseling process in the discussion of Liz's dream journals. Her interpretation of the dream material was concrete and related to the content of her life. I posed a question to her about what these dreams might mean if she viewed them from a spiritual viewpoint. Liz informed me that she was an atheist in that she did not believe in God in the traditional use of the word, but she considered herself to be a spiritual person because she believed in transformative power that was present both internally and externally. The possibility that her dreams might tap into that power was intriguing to her and one she was interested in pursuing. Over the next several weeks, as Liz explored her dreams, she was able to move beyond concrete interpretations and discover deeper meanings. Her dreams often pointed to an overwhelming fear and sense of isolation. She felt disconnected from herself and others, an interesting observation in light of her diagnosis of PTSD.

Over the course of the next several weeks, Liz continued to bring in her dream journals and short stories to share. They seemed to be a safe way to communicate about her emotions in a nonthreatening manner. I allowed her to control the content and flow of the sessions, and she tended to keep the focus on a cognitive level. Each week, in addition to dream work, we focused on the elimination of her PTSD symptoms with traditional techniques including debriefing and cognitive behavioral approaches. I also reflected feelings to her, and she tolerated them for short periods of time, moving quickly back to the cognitive, storytelling approach. As Liz became more able to tolerate experiencing uncomfortable feelings, she began to slowly reveal the traumatic events of her childhood.

Liz also began to discuss her marriage and how she was not getting the support she needed from her husband and how she never had. We discussed her difficulties with intimacy, her feelings of isolation, loneliness, and how they were related to the events of her childhood. She believed that the accident had just highlighted the reality of her life prior to it; she was alone, scared, and feeling out of control. She was able to emote and to talk about her fears, trust issues, and fears of abandonment.

Liz felt sufficiently recovered to return to work part-time. This event initially helped her to regain a sense of control and a sense of self that was familiar to her. However, it also quickly highlighted for her the differences between her public and private personae, which created anxiety and stress for her. The deficiencies in her marriage also became even more evident. She felt even more alone, isolated, and lacking support in that important relationship. She was able to connect that to the feelings she had as a child when she knew she was sick and her parents didn't believe her. We talked about that little girl and what she needed and how she could get that need met now as an adult. Again, the sessions took a spiritual tone. Liz talked about finding solace from the wise competent part of her who had survived the traumas of her life and was able to take care of her little girl.

As the anniversary of the accident approached, Liz began to experience some mild recurrence of her PTSD symptoms. We worked on how to manage the symptoms and how she might want to deal with the anniversary. She decided that a ritual to commemorate the event and the positive changes that had taken place in her life might be appropriate. The ritual held some spiritual significance for her, in that it was a way to honor the wise survivor inside of her.

In the following session, Liz reported that her mother had been diagnosed with cancer and was going to undergo surgery and chemotherapy. Despite, or perhaps because of, her mother's neglect of her during her childhood illnesses, Liz wanted to be present for her mother during this time. It seemed for her an opportunity to heal some of her own wounds. And indeed despite the pain and suffering, it was a time of healing for Liz.

One of the ways in which Liz decided to take care of her "little girl" was monthly birthday celebrations. For the first of these celebrations, she decided to give her little girl the completed painting of the black bear. She was shocked at the emotions that event evoked in her. She discussed the significance of the bear in her life. She related a story from her childhood of hearing a bear near her home and how it was comforting to her. She found a cave where it nested. In her childhood world of neglect, the bear served as a sign of hope and protection. The black bear mother was her spirit guide when she was scared and lonely. By giving it to her little girl, Liz wished for her to no longer be scared and lonely. "I know that the strength of that mother bear is in me. I am and always have been capable of taking care of myself. I can nurture the little girl until she is grown up. I can also nurture my mother now, and somehow that is healing for both of us. For the first time in my life, I feel connected to myself and to her."

Completing the painting was a significant breakthrough for Liz, but it was not the end of our work together. I continued to work with Liz as she found the strength to end a marriage that had been over for a long time. She continued to narrow the gap between her public and private personae. Despite the pain of ending her marriage and her mother's illness, Liz began to express joy and contentment in her life. She was able to be less analytical and more spontaneous. She continues to nurture her little girl and to integrate the child into the woman she has become. She is dating a man she met at work and exploring what she wants from a relationship and from her life.

## Spiritual Aspects of Liz's Journey

Liz's case clearly demonstrates that the incorporation of spirituality can be an effective intervention even with individuals who are nonreligious. In fact, Liz identified herself as an atheist. If spiritual interventions had been considered appropriate only in the context of religion, a powerful source of healing for her would have been overlooked.

The first spiritual intervention was the person-centered approach to counseling. I approached her with genuineness, unconditional positive regard, and empathic listening. I honored her fear and allowed her to control the sessions. I genuinely honored and accepted her beliefs about God. I was able to communicate that acceptance to her. We developed a genuine and trusting relationship in which she slowly began to feel safe and able to explore all the areas of her life without fear of judgment or abandonment. I heard that she was more than the sum of her PTSD symptoms. I worked with the whole of her.

The dream journal, and processing it from a spiritual perspective, was another effective spiritual intervention. In this particular circumstance, the use of a dream journal was using what was one of Liz's strengths. She liked to write, and she had vivid and powerful dreams. Dreams have long been recognized as a nonintellectual way of knowing. The spiritual interpretation of dreams can be a powerful tool in the healing process. Liz was able to understand and experience her loneliness and fear through the spiritual interpretation of her dreams. An important note is that the spiritual meaning ascribed to her dreams was always her interpretation. It is her spirit speaking, not mine.

Ritual and symbols can also be powerful spiritual interventions. Liz used ritual to deal with the anniversary of her accident and to nurture her inner child. The ritual she celebrated on the anniversary of the accident allowed her to say goodbye to some of her fears and to celebrate life. Giving her inner child the completed portrait of the black bear was a powerful ritual. The bear symbolized the strong, wise part of herself that had always been present. Completing the portrait and presenting it ritually to her inner child helped her to care for and nurture that child while recognizing and honoring the wise part of her that had always taken care of her and who would continue to do so. This event seemed to play a significant part in her life and recovery.

Perhaps the most telling aspect of the spiritual interventions is the outcome. As a result of awakening to her true nature, Liz was able to forgive her mother and actually care for her physically and emotionally. She was able to live her own life more authentically. She was able to more easily express her feelings and began to live her life less constricted by fear. She was confident in her inner wisdom and able to define her life based on her needs.

## Concluding Thoughts

Life is difficult. Helping people to overcome the difficulties of life requires that we use all of the resources at our disposal. Spirituality is a powerful resource for healing and transformation. I have discussed integrating spirituality into counseling in the context of person-centered counseling and my personal spiritual beliefs. However, I believe that spiritual interventions are appropriate, whatever the counselor's theoretical or spiritual orientation. For example, Polanski (2002) discussed the integration of spirituality from a Buddhist perspective and Adlerian theory in the helping relationship. The relationship between various spiritual approaches and other counseling theories has yet to be elucidated and is fertile ground waiting to be explored.

The integration of spirituality into the counseling process requires three elements from the counselor. First, counselors must engage in exploration of their own personal religious and spiritual beliefs and values, and their attitudes toward different beliefs and values (self-awareness). This essential step guards against imposition of the counselor's beliefs and values on clients. When considering spiritual interventions in counseling, counselors must be aware of their own motivations and possible biases. Second, the counselor must be open to learning about and accepting as valuable to the client, religious and spiritual beliefs and traditions that may be different from his or her own (knowledge). While some counselor education programs have recognized the importance of the spiritual component in helping and have incorporated spirituality into training, many have not. It is incumbent on counselors who have not received such training to educate themselves through reading, continuing education, and personal exposure to other religious and spiritual traditions. Finally, counselors must be grounded in counseling theory and explore how they can incorporate spiritual interventions that are compatible with the client's belief system into that theory (skills).

A defining criterion of counseling and what distinguishes it from other helping professions is the focus of counseling on strengths and normal human development. Spiritual development is an important aspect of overall human development and to ignore it would be a disservice to our clients and prevent us from viewing them and their lives in a holistic light.

## References

Chopra, D. (1995). *The seven spiritual laws of success.* New York: New World Library.

Das, S. Lama (1997). *Awakening the Buddha within: Tibetan wisdom for the western world.* New York: Broadway Books.

Einstein, A. (1956). *The world as I see it.* New York: Citadel Press.

Fowler, J. (1981). *Stages of faith: The psychology of human development and the quest for meaning.* San Francisco: Harper & Row.

Polanski, P. J. (2002). Exploring spiritual beliefs in relation to Adlerian theory. *Counseling and Values, 46,* 127–236.

Rogers, C. R. (1980). *A way of being.* Boston: Houghton Mifflin.

Rogers, C. R. (1961) *On becoming a person.* Boston: Houghton Mifflin.

Simpson, J. B. (1988). *Simpson's contemporary quotations.* Boston: Houghton Mifflin.

Thich, Nhat Hanh. (1995). *Living Buddha, living Christ.* New York: Riverhead Books.

# CHAPTER EIGHT

# Hear the Eagle's Cry: Native American Spiritual Traditions and Counseling

## Michael Tlanusta Garrett

> You have noticed that everything an Indian does is in a circle, and
> that is because the Power of the World always works in circles, and
> everything tries to be round. . . . The sky is round, and I have heard
> that Earth is round like a ball, and so are all the stars. The wind, in
> its greatest power, whirls. Birds make their nests in circles, for theirs
> is the same religion as ours. . . . Even the seasons form a great
> circle in their changing, and always come back again to where they
> were. The life of a person is a circle from childhood to childhood,
> and so it is in everything where power moves.
>
> —Black Elk, cited in Garrett (1998, p. 75)

The preceding quote offers a powerful glimpse into the world of Native American spirituality. With an eye toward understanding
where it is that power moves in Native spiritual traditions, this chapter
will focus on some of the following themes:

The importance of observing and listening
Lessons and perspective offered by animals and the natural environment
Ways of knowing and ways of being
Way of the Circle

Sense of connection, coexistence, and the importance of giving back
The meaning of balance
Medicine as a way of being and healing
The meaning of being a helper and caretaker
Laughter and sharing as an expression of harmony and balance

In the end, general implications will be drawn, but it is truly up to you, the reader, to draw implications that are most meaningful and useful to you in your work and personal experience. I want to thank you up front for stepping into the Native world of the Circle that will be offered here with all its beauty, challenge, and insight.

## A True Story

An Indian man stands alone staring out the window of his suburban apartment with a .45 caliber handgun pointed at his head. He is in his thirties now and has battled alcoholism for years. He has fought to be a good single father to his two young sons. He has grappled with that emptiness deep down in his spirit all his life, and that constant nagging urge to always take just one more drink. He has been in and out of treatment programs, on and off with AA, and now he just wants all the pain to stop. He can feel the coldness of the barrel against his throbbing temple, and as he stares out of the window at the beautiful summer day unfolding before him, he notices a little turtle struggling to go from one place to another. Then he notices the cat crouched not far away from the turtle waiting for the right moment to pounce on its helpless prey. The turtle, spying the cat in waiting, quickly pulls into its shell. Just then, the cat leaps toward the turtle, pawing and hissing.

Safely in its shell, the turtle remains unharmed by the persistent cat that tries to open this troublesome package, knocking it upside down, prying, but to no avail. Frustrated, the cat wanders off in search of easier prey. Moments pass before the turtle emerges slowly from the safety of its shell once again. First the head, then a leg or two, and finally everything back where it was. The turtle, which is lying upside down from the ordeal, slowly pushes himself with one leg, flips himself back right side up, and continues on his journey.

The Indian man, who has become so engrossed in this drama unfolding before him, has lowered the gun from his head as he continues to watch. The turtle comes to a log. The man looks on, expecting the turtle to find some way to go around this barrier, but the turtle just slowly, patiently climbs over the log and flips down on the other side of it. As the man glances down at the gun in his hand, the wetness in his eyes swells. As he looks back out the window, the turtle has disappeared (Garrett & Carroll, 2000).

The preceding true story happened to a friend of mine, and reminds me of so many true stories of Native people who struggle to live life just as everyone does in a world rich with meaning and messages of truth, but also full of distractions and limiting barriers. In desperation, my friend was inadvertently asking himself that question—what is life— but didn't have an answer, or so he thought. The story reminds me of an old quote by a Native leader named Crowfoot who pondered: "What is life? It is the flash of a firefly in the night. It is the breath of a buffalo in the wintertime. It is the little shadow which runs across the grass and loses itself in the sunset" (Crowfoot, cited in Padilla, 1994, p. 11). Perhaps the simplest forms of beauty are also the most powerful. Could it be that life is as simple as the beauty contained within the smile of a small child, or the torrid glow of someone in love?

## Observing and Listening

The importance of observing and listening in the traditional approach to Native spirituality includes paying attention to and reflecting on the lessons offered by our relatives in the animal world. Therein lies powerful Medicine that guides any person on his or her life-journey. One such lesson comes from considering the difference between Hawk and Eagle:

> When hunting, Hawk sees Mouse . . . and dives directly for it. When hunting, Eagle sees the whole pattern . . . sees movement in the general pattern . . . and dives for the movement, learning only later that it is Mouse.   (Spencer, 1990, p. 17)

The difference between Hawk and Eagle teaches Native Americans the difference between Specificity and Wholeness. All things are connected, and all things are constantly in motion, just as the energy of life is constantly moving and changing. Wholeness shows us the motion of all things, and Specificity gives us a point of reference from which to view all things by reminding us of "relation" or relationship between one thing and another. Through Eagle, Native people are reminded of the great expanse of the universe and its circular motion of interconnectedness and interdependence, remembering always to keep the larger picture in view as they move through life. Through Hawk, Native people are reminded of the need to remember where they are in relation to everything else, focusing neither completely on themselves nor on everything else, but rather recognizing the relationship that exists and honoring that relationship at all times (Garrett, 1996).

Taking the time to consider the relationships and meanings of our brothers and sisters in the animal world is one example of the Native approach to spiritual learning as an attempt is made to replace wanting with giving.

## A Way of Knowing

One of my students said about my teaching, "There are many professors, but few teachers. You are truly a teacher. You are the only teacher who has taught me from the inside-out as opposed to the outside-in. You have helped me find my truth and know my own intelligence. . . ." This quote best illustrates my philosophy of both teaching and counseling through a focus on growth with the deepest belief that true learning happens from the inside-out. You know that you have learned something when you can really feel it and make a connection of some kind, even long after that moment it was learned. True learning continues uninterrupted, oblivious to time.

I have thought about this quote many times since it was said to me in 1997, when I was a young assistant professor in my first faculty position. When I think about my philosophy of teaching and counseling, I wonder how it came to be. I see, in my mind, all the many teachers and counselors in my life who lived what they professed to be true and never approached learning as being more important than relationships as a form of connection and true learning in itself. True learning is relational and forming connections is the highest form of learning. I think about the essence of Native spirituality, so difficult to define, so pervasively exploited in our mainstream culture, and so deeply rooted and sacred to the people for whom it means everything, not just a way of life and knowing, but as life itself.

When I was younger, and people would ask me, what is Indian Medicine, or what is your religion, or what is Native spirituality, I used to struggle picking just the right words, in just the right way to best describe something that meant so much in my life and to the survival of my family over generations. Always, I walked away feeling that I had not done the concept, the practices, the experience very much justice at all. These days, I am older and fortunate to have become a father. I have given it the same amount of thought as I anticipate teaching my son all the things that I was taught by the many teachers I have had over time. Now, when asked, "What is Native spirituality," I simply say, it is a feeling. It is a breath of life that moves through you somehow, and just is what it needs to be at any given point in time.

As you read my words here, it is important for you to know who I am. I am an enrolled member of the Eastern Band of Cherokee and the son of an Eastern Band of the Cherokee enrolled tribal member from western North Carolina and his wife, who is German by heritage, daughter of a Methodist minister and his wife from Ohio. My mother and father met quite by chance, or so it might seem, one summer when my mother was a young seventeen-year-old cashier at one of the tourist shops on the reservation and my father was a twenty-one-year-old local college student. As the story goes, he walked into the laundromat late one evening and encountered my mother there, doing her laundry. In a clumsy attempt to start up conversation with this striking young woman, he perched himself up on one of the old washers, crossed his legs, and introduced himself, saying, "You can tell that I'm Indian because I'm sitting Indian style." My mother, who had a steady high school boyfriend back home, was less than impressed with this underweight but persistent Native guy. But at the urging of a common friend who showed up that night, my mother and father ended up taking a short drive to have cokes together, then a longer drive that was intended to have taken my mother home, but rather, took them high into the Blue Ridge Parkway. There, in the dead of night, my father reached his arm over as if he were going to make a move on the young woman. Much to her relief, she started for the car door only to find that my father was reaching into the back seat to pull out his guitar with which he serenaded her for four hours. As I am told, it was pure love from there, and the rest is history, although not all of it easy.

Shortly after meeting my mother, my father was drafted into the Navy during the Vietnam war, and was fortunate to survive his tour of duty, during which a beautiful baby boy was born. Subsequently, he left the military to go into industry and we moved many, many times, while he put himself through graduate school to obtain his doctorate in public health education. Still, we always returned to the reservation from which my father came, and I spent most of my time there growing up. The beauty of the natural environment there in the mountains of western North Carolina was always a given, and you never thought twice about it until you had to leave it, which we did when I was fifteen years old. My mother's spiritual tradition, coming from poor German, Methodist, farming families in rural Ohio, gave her a sense of pride in and loyalty to family and what it means to work hard to survive in this world. My father's spiritual tradition, coming from a poor Cherokee family in the mountains of western North Carolina gave him a deep respect for and connection with the natural surroundings, with ceremony, and with family. Influenced by the values of these spiritual traditions, but raised primarily in my father's cultural tradition and beliefs, my upbringing taught me how important it was to respect the culture and customs of your people, to respect and learn from the natural environment, to value family, to look for meaning in every experience that comes your way, both good and bad, to seek harmony and balance in life, to maintain your peace, and to listen to your heart.

When I think about who I am and where I am in life now, I think about the fact that I come from people who care about people and value life. I became a counselor for a number of reasons, but partly because tribal scholarship and family support allowed me to choose something that I really loved and was passionate about. My training as a counselor and counselor-educator involved more time than I can count on theories of change and development, based on the philosophies, beliefs, and experiences of white men. That never bothered me, especially because I am part white. However, I did always make it a point to remember where I came from, and that the philosophies, beliefs, and experiences of Native people were no less valuable, powerful, or true. To this day, I have tried to integrate both my professional training and my personal background as a Native person into my writing, research, and practice. I invite you to consider the very simple ways of Native life that I call the Way of the Circle as a guide for both personal and professional practice.

## The Way of the Circle

When you first arise in the morning, give thanks to the Creator (Great Spirit, Great One, Great Creator), to the Four Directions, Mother Earth, Father Sky, all of our relations, for the life within you, and for all the life around you.

All things are connected.

Remember that all things have purpose, everything has its place.

Honor others by treating them with kindness and consideration; always assume that a guest is tired, cold, and hungry, making sure to provide him or her with the best of what you have to offer.

If you have more than you need for yourself and your family, consider performing a "giveaway" by distributing your possessions to others who are in need.

You are bound by your word that cannot be broken except by permission of the other party.

Seek harmony and balance in all things.

It is always important to remember where you are in relation to everything else, and to contribute to the Circle in whatever way you can.

Sharing is the best part of receiving.

Practice silence and patience in all things as a reflection of self-control, endurance, dignity, reverence, and inner calm.

Practice modesty in all things; avoid boasting and loud behavior that attracts attention to yourself.

Know the things that contribute to your well-being, and those things that lead to your destruction.

Always ask permission, and give something for everything that is received, including giving thanks and honoring all living things.

Be aware of what is around you, what is inside of you, and always show respect: Treat every person with respect, from the tiniest child to the oldest elder.

Do not stare at others; drop your eyes as a sign of respect, especially in the presence of elders, teachers, or community leaders.

Always give a sign of greeting when passing a friend or stranger.

Never criticize or talk about someone in a harmful, negative way.

Never touch something that belongs to someone else without permission.

Respect the privacy of every person, making sure to never intrude upon someone's quiet moments or personal space.

Never interfere in the affairs of another by asking questions or offering advice.

Never interrupt others.

In another person's home, follow his or her customs rather than your own.

Treat with respect all things held sacred to others whether you understand them or not.

Treat the Earth as your mother, give to her, protect her, honor her; show deep respect for the animal world, plant world, and mineral world.

Listen to guidance offered by all of your surroundings; expect this guidance to come in the form of prayer, dreams, quiet solitude, and in the words and deeds of wise elders and friends.

Listen with your heart.

Learn from your experiences, and always be open to new ones.

Always remember that a smile is something sacred, to be shared.

Live each day as it comes.

In my family, grandparents have helped children learn a right way to live life through stories, quiet observation, and listening with both mind and heart for generations and generations. Within Native spirituality, this serves as a set of unspoken rules across tribal lines for how one is to act in this world in order to respect the gift of life, and to move through this world learning what one is here to learn and contribute. These rules are not written down anywhere, and often are learned very much through experience and observation. For all intents and purposes, these unspoken rules don't even really have a name, so we could call them the "Indian commandments," but in order to capture the true essence, we will just call them the Way of the Circle (Garrett, 1996; Lake, 1991) and they serve as the foundation for Native spirituality.

## Native Spirituality

In the traditional way, Native American elders are honored as highly respected persons due to the lifetime's worth of wisdom they have acquired through continuous experience. Elders bear an important responsibility for the tribal community by functioning as parents, teachers, community leaders, and spiritual guides. Referring to an elder as Grandmother, Grandfather, Uncle, or Aunt is to refer to a very special relationship that exists with that elder through deep respect and admiration. To use these terms and other more general terms such as "old woman" or "old man" greatly honors someone who has achieved the status of elder (Garrett & Garrett, 1997).

Elders have responsibility for directing children's attention to the things with which they co-exist (family, community, trees, plants, rocks, animals, elements, the land) and to the meaning of these things. In this way, Native American children develop a heightened level of sensitivity for all of the relationships of which they are a part, and which are a part of them, for the circular (cyclical) motion of life, and for the customs and traditions of their people. Raising a child is considered one of the most important responsibilities with which a person can be blessed. For many tribes, a child is viewed as a sacred gift from the Creator, and therefore as more of a pleasure than an obligation or burden. The participation of aunts, uncles, brothers, sisters, and valued friends in the raising of and caring for a child adds emphasis to the sense of unity reflected in relationships.

There is a very special kind of relationship based on mutual respect and caring between Indian elders and Indian children as one moves through the "life circle" from *being cared for* to *caring for* (Red Horse, 1997). With increase in age comes an increase in the sacred responsibility to family, clan, and tribe. Native American elders have the opportunity to relate to the children the tradition that their life force carries the spirits of their ancestors. With such an emphasis on connectedness, children are a focal point in Native American culture, as illustrated by the following anecdote:

> In a conversation with his aging grandfather, a young Indian man asked, "Grandfather, what is the purpose of life?" After a long time in thought, the old man looked up and said, "Grandson, children are the purpose of life. We were once children and someone cared for us, and now it is our time to care." (from Brendtro, Brokenleg & Van Bockern, 1990, p. 45)

The traditional approach to relationship focuses on a sense of connectedness, thankfulness, and the importance of giving back. Many Native American children learn to perceive Native American elders, the keepers of the sacred ways, as protectors, mentors, teachers, and support-givers. Meanwhile, Native American elders, whose primary purpose is to care for and guide the children, are reminded of the spirit of playfulness, innocence, and curiosity through the realization that there is always something to learn and always something to appreciate.

Sometimes, I think about my grandfather. He died when I was eight. People tell me that I look like him, but it has been so long now, I have a hard time remembering what he looked like exactly. I have a picture of him standing outside a gas station somewhere in Arizona, smirking to himself as he is walking out the door because it was smaller than his tiny gas station back home on the reservation. Sometimes, I wonder, does his spirit dwell with me?

I remember the way he smelled. I remember his quiet, pensive stare, as though he were able to transport himself so far into other worlds and see things more clearly than most people ever do in any lifetime. He seldom said much, but rather let his actions speak for him. He was a World War Two Navy veteran, survivor of Pearl Harbor, champion boxer, husband, father, and TV repairman who worked himself to the bone. He had a dream inside him I think, but I don't know what it was for sure. I always knew I was safe with him. Though not a large man, he emanated strength of both body and of resolve. He had a gentle, kind way about him that made people around the reservation respect him a great deal, knowing that he would, and did, do anything he could for someone in need. He understood what it meant to suffer. His father died at age twenty-seven of a massive heart attack, leaving my grandfather, the oldest of two brothers to take care of the family. Like so many of his generation, he lied about his age to get into the Navy so he could make a living in order to bring home an income for his family. I remember his dark piercing eyes, and leathery, brown face—an old man from the mountains and an old sailor. I can remember his strong, thin, scarred hands.

When my son was born, I wondered if my grandfather helped carry him into this world. The week before, I remembered having a dream of my grandfather walking hand in hand with a little boy from some distant place. The day of delivery, while walking in a stairwell to calm my nerves a little before our son was to be born, I felt a presence brush past me. It felt like something familiar, but I just couldn't put my finger on it, although it somehow put me at ease. I hadn't slept in two days, and had been afraid for my wife and my soon-to-be-born child. I immediately returned to the delivery room where the doctor was preparing to help my wife give birth. With complications, my son was born at 2:30 P.M. on May 8, 2003, and it was the scariest, yet most moving experience I have ever had. Not long after delivery, someone said to me, "Did you realize that today is your grandpa's birthday?"

The other day, someone told me that my son looks like my grandfather. That old, familiar picture of my grandfather walking out of that tiny gas station in Arizona lingers above my son's crib among other family objects. Time flows like rivers, but love never dies.

## Balance and Harmony: Walking in Step

Balance in Native spirituality is a desired state wherein one is in harmony with the universe, walking in step with the natural way (flow) of things. Being in harmony means being in step with the universe and with its sacred rhythms. This is what many Native people refer to as "Good Medicine." By contrast, being in disharmony or "dis-ease" means being out of step with the universe and its sacred rhythms. This invites illness. Disharmony results when we are out of balance, our energies are unfocused or poorly focused, and we lose sight of our place in the universe. Well-being occurs when we seek and find our unique place in the universe and experience the continuous cycle of receiving and giving through respect and reverence for the beauty of all living things. Thus, the wellness of the mind, body, spirit, and natural environment are an expression of the proper balance in the relationship of all things. If one disturbs or disrupts the natural balance, illness or dis-ease in any of these four areas may be the result. This is one of the primary reasons for keeping one's life energy strong and clear in relation to others and to the natural environment.

Native languages are an interesting measure of what is valued in the culture and in what way. In many Native American languages, there is no word for "religion" because spiritual practices are an integral part of every aspect of daily life. They are necessary for the harmony and balance, or wellness, of the individual, family, clan, and community. Healing and worship are considered one and the same. For many Native American people, the concept of health and wellness is not only a physical state, but also a spiritual one. In addition, the focus of Native spirituality emphasizes a spatial reality rather than a linear one (Deloria, 1994). In a linear reality, the focus is on select people and events occurring over the course of a linear past, present, and future. In a spatial reality, the focus is on the relationship that people have with their surroundings and the spiritual power and meaning held within specific places in the environment rather than events and/or people. Thus, a Native approach to spirituality focuses on relation and connection with the truths that exist within and around oneself.

Different Native tribal languages have different ways of expressing the idea of honoring one's sense of connection, but the meaning is similar across nations referring to the belief that human beings exist on Mother Earth to be helpers and protectors of life. In Native communities, it is not uncommon to hear people use the term *caretaker* in some form or another. From the perspective of a traditionalist, to see one's purpose as that of caretaker is to accept responsibility for the gift of life by taking good care of that gift, the gift of life that others have received, and the surrounding beauty of the world in which we live (Garrett & Wilbur, 1999). More or less, the essence of Native American spirituality is about "feeling" that sense of connection that comes in many ways (Wilbur, 1999a, 1999b). Although there are differences between individuals and across nations, it is possible to generalize to some extent about a number of basic beliefs characterizing Native American traditionalism and spirituality. The following, adapted from Locust (1988, pp. 317–18), elaborates on a number of basic Native American spiritual and traditional beliefs:

1. There is a single higher power known as Creator, Great Creator, Great Spirit, or Great One, among other names (this being is sometimes referred to in gender form, but does not necessarily exist as one particular gender or another). There are also lesser beings known as spirit beings or spirit helpers.

2. Plants and animals, like humans, are part of the spirit world. The spirit world exists side by side with, and intermingles with, the physical world. Moreover, the spirit existed in the spirit world before it came into a physical body and will exist after the body dies.

3. Human beings are made up of a spirit, mind, and body. The mind, body, and spirit are all interconnected; therefore, illness affects the mind and spirit as well as the body.

4. Wellness is harmony in body, mind, and spirit; unwellness is disharmony in mind, body, and spirit.

5. Natural unwellness is caused by the violation of a sacred social or natural law of Creation (such as participating in a sacred ceremony while under the influence of alcohol or drugs, or having had sex within four days of the ceremony).

6. Unnatural unwellness is caused by conjuring (or witchcraft) from those with destructive intentions.

7. Each of us is responsible for our own wellness by keeping ourselves attuned to self, relations, environment, and universe.

This list of beliefs crosses tribal boundaries, but is by no means comprehensive. It does, however, provide insight into some of the assumptions that may be held by traditional Native spirituality.

Understanding Native spiritual traditions means understanding the direction of one's path as a caretaker moving to the rhythm of the sacred heartbeat. The constant seeking for balance and harmony in life mirrors that constant movement in nature. No symbol in Native traditions captures life, love, and the pursuit of harmony better than the Eagle feather and the circle as sacred representations across tribal nations of striving for harmony and balance.

## Enter the Circle

Metaphorically, as one steps into a worldview encompassed by the traditional Native Circle, it becomes easier to understand how one orients oneself mentally, physically, spiritually, and spatially; how one becomes aware of energy within oneself and around oneself as a source of power; how to use that essence of energy in the context of relation; and the necessity of opening oneself to the guiding principles of a personal vision that directs us toward our purpose in the Circle.

**Honoring Our Truths.**   In order to better understand a Native worldview, it is necessary to consider some of the underlying values that permeate a Native worldview and existence. Some of these values include the importance of community contribution, sharing, acceptance, cooperation, harmony and balance, noninterference, extended family, attention to nature, immediacy of time, awareness of the relationship, and a deep respect for elders (Garrett, 1999). All in all, these traditional Native values show the importance of honoring, through harmony and balance, what is believed to be a very sacred connection with the energy of life, and thus plays an important role in the way traditional Native ceremonies are conducted.

**Calling to the Four Winds.** Traditionally, it is believed that each of the Four Directions in the Circle represent one of the four winds and/or the elements found within nature. This is a useful concept in better understanding the traditional Native American emphasis on harmony and balance of mind, body, spirit, and natural environment. The following example drawn from traditional Cherokee teachings (Garrett & Garrett, 1996; Garrett, 1998) as well as the work of Brendtro, Brokenleg, and Van Bockern (1990) describes each of the directions comprising the harmony and balance of the inner circle:

| | |
|---|---|
| East (belonging): | Where do you belong (or not belong); who's your family/clan/tribe? |
| South (mastery): | What do you do well; what do you enjoy doing? |
| West (independence): | What are your (sources of) strengths; what limits you? |
| North (generosity): | What do you have to offer; what do you receive? |

From a traditional Native perspective, as you seek to answer these questions within yourself, you come into a different level of awareness about your own unique Medicine, harmony and balance, unique challenges and life lessons, and needs for healing.

**Circles Within Circles.** Life, from a traditional Native perspective, is viewed as a series of concentric circles that emanate from one another like the rippling waters of a lake (Garrett, 1998). The first circle is the inner circle, representing that which is within us, being our spirit, the culmination of all of our experiences and the power that comes from the very essence of our being. The next circle is family/clan. Family might be blood relations, and it might be family of choice or adopted family (family in spirit); this circle also includes tribe/nation/community, since this is the social context in which we live and represents a different sense of belonging. The third circle is the natural environment, Mother Earth, and all our relations. A fourth and final circle consists of the spirit world that encompasses all of the other circles, and is believed to be where the Creator dwells, along with all our ancestors and other spirit helpers/guides. Therefore, circles of life energy surround us, exist within us, and make up the many relationships of our existence. In all, we each have a circle of self, comprised of the many facets of our own development (such as mind, body, spirit, and natural surroundings); a circle of immediate family, extended family, tribal family, community, and nation; a circle consisting of all our relations in the natural environment; and a circle of our universal surroundings (Garrett & Myers, 1996).

**Taking Your Medicine.**    In Native tradition, one experiences life through the senses, and it is through one's emotional experience of life that one becomes aware of "Medicine." In the traditional Native way, Medicine can consist of physical remedies such as herbs, teas, or poultices to treat physical ailments, but Medicine is also the very essence of a person's inner being. It is that which gives a person inner power (Garrett & Garrett, 1996). Medicine is in every tree, plant, rock, animal, and person. It is in the light, the soil, the water, and the wind. Medicine is something that happened ten years ago that still makes a person smile when thinking about it. Medicine is that old friend who calls up out of the blue just because she wanted to. There is Medicine in watching a small child play. Medicine is in the reassuring smile of an elder. There is Medicine is every event, memory, place, person, and movement. There is even Medicine in "empty space" if one knows how to use it. And there can be powerful Medicine in painful or hurtful experiences. Even such experiences offer the opportunity to see more clearly the way things connect and disconnect in the greater flow of this stream called life.

**Connect/Disconnect.**    Central to Native traditions is the importance of "relation" as a total way of existing in the world. The concept of family extends to brothers and sisters in the animal world, the plant world, the mineral world, Mother Earth, Father Sky, and so on. The power of relation is symbolized by the Circle of Life (sometimes referred to as the Web of Life), so commonly represented throughout the customs, traditions, and art forms of Native people (Dufrene, 1990). The Circle thus reflects not only the interrelationship of all living beings, but the natural progression or growth of life itself. Harmony and balance are necessary for the survival of all life. Thus, *proper relations* or giving thanks to *all our* *relations* are common phrases in Indian country. In the context of daily life and ceremonial practice, *proper relations* means learning how to connect with certain constructive or creative forces, and disconnect from destructive forces. This means learning about one's own harmony and balance in the framework of the circles in which a person exists.

**Through Eagle's Eyes.** From a traditional Native perspective, it is important throughout life to either seek your vision or continue honoring your vision. In Native tradition, vision is an inner knowledge of your own Medicine and purpose in the Greater Circle revealed to you through your spirit helpers (Garrett & Garrett, 1996). This means connecting with your inner power and opening yourself to the guidance of the spirits. This may happen in ceremony, or it may happen in other ways such as through dreams, particular signs, animal messengers, or certain experiences/events that come your way for a reason. Understanding one's vision is understanding the direction of one's path as a caretaker, moving to the rhythm of the sacred heartbeat through the experience of all that is sacred in life and ceremony.

**Remembering the Circle**

Traditional Native peoples view all things as having spiritual energy and importance as a way of seeing all of life reflected in each living thing. All things are connected, all things have life, and all things are worthy of respect and reverence. Spiritual "being" essentially requires only that individuals seek their place in the universe. Everything else will follow in good time. Because everything was created with a specific purpose to fulfill, no one should have the power to interfere with or to impose upon others which path is the best to follow (Good Tracks, 1973). In order to better understand what it means to "walk in step" according to Native American spirituality, one can remember the following four Native principles (Garrett & Wilbur, 1999) as a general rule of thumb for living in harmony and balance:

1. Everything is alive.
2. Everything has purpose.
3. All things are connected.
4. Embrace the Medicine of every living being to embrace your vision.

In Cherokee teachings, every living being possesses an inner power referred to as "Medicine," or way of life, which connects us to all other living beings through the heart. However, if we fail to respect our relations (with all living beings, the Creator, Mother Earth, ourselves, and the Four

Directions) and to keep ourselves in step with the universe, we invite illness by falling out of harmony and balance, much like a dancer failing
to move in step with the rhythm of the drum. A person's Medicine is
his or her power, and it can be used for creative purposes or destructive
purposes—either contributing to or taking away from the Greater Circle
of Life. Being in harmony means "being in step with the universe." Being
in disharmony means "being out-of-step with the universe." As helpers
and caretakers, we are constantly challenged to seek our own harmony
and balance in the Circle as we seek to help others do the same.

## Caretaker

> I'm the spirit's janitor. All I do is wipe the windows a little bit so you
> can see out for yourself.    (Garrett, 1998, p. 145)

By stepping into the role of a helper and caretaker, all of this life is
looked upon as a sacred gift from the Creator to be treated always with
reverence and great care. The traditional way of life is based on a very
basic set of principles involving demonstration of respect for oneself,
one's relatives or "relations" (all living creatures), Mother Earth, and
those in the spirit world. Interestingly, it is not only human beings that
can be helpers, as we soon discover when we, as helpers, draw upon the
healing and many lessons offered by all living beings in our surroundings. These very basic beliefs and traditions can serve as valuable lessons
working with people in therapeutic contexts.

## Call of the Owl: Case Scenario

Jayne is a fifty-one-year-old, divorced, Native woman who was referred to
counseling for mild depression and anxiety resulting from "family issues."
She is an enrolled member of her tribe, and grew up on the reservation
where she still resides today. Currently, Jayne works in the human resource department of a casino owned and operated by her tribe. Jayne
has been described as a tireless worker who often puts the needs of her
job ahead of herself and her family. This hard-working attitude has
allowed her to advance in the ranks from a secretarial position to the
managerial level in which she is currently working. She is very happy
with her career and looks forward to retiring in fifteen more years in
addition to finally paying off her home. Jayne admits that her life hasn't
all been easy, and that although she tries to get along with everyone,

there are people in and around the reservation who resent her having become so successful in a short period of time.

Both of Jayne's parents are Native. Her mother is "still traditional" although she was put through Catholic boarding school and never talks about the experience. Her father, who was mixed, and now deceased, managed to pass for white and worked as a laborer from the time that he was twelve years old. According to Jayne, the fact that she also is of mixed background has caused her some trouble throughout her life with some of the full-bloods who live on the reservation. She says that it bothered her more when she was young, but now she just does what she needs to do and doesn't worry too much about what other people think of her. Jayne was born on the reservation, as were her older brother and sister, and has lived there pretty much all her life.

Jayne originally wanted to study to be a nurse and did go to community college for a while where she did exceptionally well. After the first year, however, she eloped with her boyfriend and they had a house built on the reservation through tribal housing. Jayne and her husband had their first child a year and a half later. Their second child was born three years after that. Both she and her husband worked from the time that the children were young while other family members kept them. Jayne and her husband were married for fifteen years before "his jealousy" finally got to her, and they ended up in divorce. He moved out, and she and the children then lived in the house by themselves.

Now, her children are grown and have left home. The oldest has married and started a family. The youngest is attending school on a tribal scholarship in a nearby metropolitan area. Although Jayne has dated periodically since her divorce, nothing really serious ever came of it. She has pretty much lived by herself and "gotten used to it." In the absence of marital ties, Jayne threw herself into her work, at first out of necessity to support her children, and later out of a deep sense of pride and accomplishment that it gave her.

The only real hobby that Jayne enjoys is beadwork, which she used to do more often when she was younger. Now, she seldom has enough extra time to sit down with it and often finds herself getting pulled in other directions. However, she does still take great pride in her beadwork, and has won a number of local and regional awards for it. She looks forward to putting her beadwork skills back to use for her oldest granddaughter who is learning to dance and is in need of regalia.

For the past three years, Jayne has struggled with mild depression and anxiety. It began when she found out that her older sister had cancer. Whatever time Jayne was not working or spending with her granddaughters,

Jayne has been taking care of her sister in whatever way she can. She says that she really has not thought about the possibility that her sister could die because she couldn't imagine life without her. Recently though, on a number of occasions, she has heard Ugugu (owl) in the early morning, and although she isn't superstitious, she can't help but being in a panic now.

## Medicine Way: Implications for Practice

A number of questions for consideration might be posed in thinking through some important implications with this case:

What is the purpose of life for Jayne, and what gives her life purpose?
In what ways has Jayne reevaluated her own life and relationships since finding out about her sister's illness?
To what does Jayne attribute her sister's illness?
What has it meant to Jayne to go from "being cared for" to "caring for," that is, daughter to mother to grandmother?
Who will care for Jayne when she most needs it?
What does the owl mean both in Jayne's culture and for her personally? What might the owl be saying to her?
What does it mean to Jayne to be Native and an enrolled member of her nation/tribe?
What do Jayne's spiritual beliefs and traditions consist of?
Where does Jayne feel the most and least connected?
What role does harmony and balance play in Jayne's life and where does she find the most peace?
Where does Jayne find healing?

These questions are suggested to stimulate thought on how to proceed with the case based on concepts of Native spirituality, but they also could serve as process questions in actual work with this client. Naturally, her answers to any one of these could lead to further exploration. For example, if she says more about the conflict between the traditional beliefs with which she was raised and some of the more assimilated beliefs she has espoused over the years, counseling could be directed toward reconciling that conflict, helping Jayne experience less dissonance and working toward meaningful insights and personal peace.

As counselors, we have the responsibility and privilege of being able to serve as facilitators and guides for our clients as they walk their own Medicine path and seek their own vision. Archie Fire Lame Deer, Lakota Medicine Man, described the role of such a guide: "To be a Medicine person, you have to experience everything, live life to the fullest. If you don't experience the human side of everything, how can you help teach or heal? To be a good Medicine person, you've got to be humble. You've got to be lower than a worm and higher than an eagle" (cited in Garrett, 1998, p. 41).

The case scenario and working questions presented above may stimulate reflection about Native spirituality and the many forms it might take in people's lives and in therapeutic work. Though it is not our job to be a Medicine person in the Native traditional sense of healing, it does seem that we, as counselors, walk a parallel path as another form of helper (Matheson, 1996). One wonders, as we reflect on Native American spirituality, about the question that my great-grandfather posed to my father many times when he was being a stubborn, inquisitive little boy: "Does the worm live in the ground, or does the worm fly in the sky?" Perhaps that is a question we should ask ourselves when we are working with our clients. Perhaps that is a question we should ask ourselves the next time we see a turtle walking its journey unimpeded, the smile of a little giggling baby chattering to some unknown companion standing close, the dance of the hawk upon invisible winds, or hear the cry of the Eagle in our hearts and in our minds. It may be true that everything has a certain place in the Greater Circle. Maybe that is what makes life so worth living as we fulfill our purpose of discovering that which is true, sometimes, over and over again, and experience all that is sacred as we learn to care-take and "take care."

In terms of applying Native spiritual beliefs and traditions to therapeutic settings with Native and non-Native clients alike, there are a number of important considerations. On the one hand, therapeutic techniques that draw on Native traditions can be useful combinations of age-old wisdom with contemporary practice (see, for example, Garrett, 2002; Garrett & Crutchfield, 1997; Garrett & Garrett, 2002; Garrett, Garrett & Brotherton, 2001; Roberts-Wilbur, Wilbur, Garrett & Yuhas, 2001 for further information on the use of Native-based techniques and practices in therapeutic settings). On the other hand, a more formalized implementation of Native ceremony could also be useful, depending on a number of factors, including how the ceremony is conducted, for what purpose, who participates, where the ceremony is conducted, and who conducts it.

Across tribal nations, there are many different ceremonies used for healing, giving thanks, celebrating, clearing the way, and blessing (Garrett & Garrett, 2002). The underlying goal of these ceremonies, from a Native perspective, is almost always to offer thanks for, create, and maintain a strong sense of connection through harmony and balance of mind, body, and spirit with the natural environment. From a Native perspective, the main purpose of such healing ceremonies is to "keep oneself in good relations." This can mean honoring or healing a connection with oneself, between oneself and others (relationships, that is, family, friends, community), between oneself and the natural environment, or between oneself and the spirit world. Sometimes, healing ceremonies involve all of these. Among the various traditions of healing ceremonies utilized by Native people, a few more well-known examples include sweat lodge, vision quest, clearing-way ceremony, blessing-way ceremony, pipe ceremony, sunrise ceremony, sundance, powwow, and countless others. One of the functions of ceremonial practice through the group is to reaffirm one's connection with that which is sacred.

One possible approach for more widespread use of Native spirituality in counseling practice is to combine individual or group counseling with cultural technique, while leaving some of the more sacred, tribally specific, ceremonial aspects out of the process. All in all, adjustments can be made to utilize an adaptation of a very traditional and sacred cultural practice with great therapeutic benefits for clients, while maintaining a deep sense of respect and reverence for the traditions from which it comes. Always keep in mind, the true purpose of ceremony is to provide a way for people to give back, in thanks for all the things they receive, and to create an openness of spirit that makes life the growing, interconnected experience it is meant to be from a traditional Native perspective.

## Laughing It Up: The Most Important Ingredient of Healing?

As a final thought to the discussion of implications for practice, I would be remiss to leave out a thought or two on the cultural value placed on humor by Native people, and its power to invoke healing. Contrary to the stereotypical belief that Indian people are solemn, stoic figures poised against a backdrop of tepees, tomahawks, and headdresses, the fact is, Native people love to laugh (Maples, Dupey, Torres-Rivera, Phan, Vereen & Garrett, 2001). Indeed, it is a critical part of the culture and spiritual tradition.

Mealtime, for many Native people, is one of many sacred places where humor seems to work its magic. It is amazing to watch the transformation that occurs when people come together around food, and really begin to open up. In Indian country, mealtime is sometimes the worst time to try to eat because everyone is laughing, cutting up, sharing side-splitting stories, and teasing each other.

I remember once being invited to participate in a Navajo healing cere-mony for a woman, while visiting the Navajo reservation. As is true for many tribes, there are so many between-group differences, not the least of which is language, that I did not know what to expect. As we respect-fully entered the low, earth-bound entrance to the traditional Hogan, we found silence among a number of family members already inside. A very old Navajo Medicine Man seemed to be mentally preparing himself in one corner as he put his things in place. Next to him sat an old woman, sitting calmly with eyes down, gathering herself for the ceremony. As we sat there together sensing one another and warming-up, I felt my-self becoming a little uneasy because I did not know their ceremonies, language, songs, or "rules."

The old woman said something to the others in Navajo, and every-one proceeded to get some of the food that was laid out there along one of the sides. As we sat together eating, there was much conversation in Navajo and laughter about one thing or another. A friend said to me, "My grandmother wants to know where you and your people are from." I told her North Carolina, and she sat there for a moment pensive. Then, the old woman uttered a few words, and my friend translated for me that the grandmother mentioned that I was the man from the land beneath the sun and she had never been there, but heard that they had a lot more water there. That phrase, "from the land beneath the sun," really struck me, and as I sat there considering its beauty and power, another guy spoke to me directly in English. "So you got your Ph.D., huh?" I told him yes, being careful not to be boastful in the company of my generous hosts, and he said, "Yeah, me too." I looked at the man, who was very modestly dressed, had a few teeth missing, and didn't at all look like someone who had finished a terminal degree. Then, he burst out, "post-hole digger," slapping me in the back and laughing uncon-trollably. At that point, I had been designated razzable (teasable) and therefore okay. The ceremony began not long after we finished our meal. Except for listening to my father's old chants, especially sung to my little boy, I have never heard anything so beautiful and so moving since that time, as the vision and sound of that old Medicine Man singing his powerful healing song for four straight hours, inviting the healing spirits to come into our space and help a woman and her family.

Another way that humor finds a way to work its magic in Native tra-ditions is through the many stories and legends that have been passed down for generations from elders to children. Many tribal oral traditions emphasize important life lessons through the subtle humor expressed in these stories. Frequently, it is the arrogant, manipulative, vain, clownlike figure of Rabbit, Possum, Coyote, or Raven that learns a hard lesson in humility, much to the amusement of others (Herring, 1994). Native people understand that laughter plays a very important role in the continued survival of the tribal communities, and it is an unspoken foundation of the culture. After all, laughter relieves stress and creates an atmosphere of sharing and connectedness. In essence, humor and the sharing of laughter through stories, legends, and other means may be one of the truer forms of balance and harmony as people come together with a sense of community and belonging. As George Good Striker, Blackfoot elder, puts it, "Humor is the WD-40 of healing" (cited in Garrett, 1998, p. 137).

## Down by the River: Another True Story

This true story is one that my father has told me many times, and somehow holds a special place in my heart as I imagine my father as a little boy down by the Oconaluftee River with his grandfather.

"Some of my fondest memories of when I was still a little one go back to times spent with my grandfather, Oscar Rogers, who was Eastern Cherokee. We would spend time sitting on the rocks by the Oconaluftee River in Cherokee, North Carolina. 'What do you see when you look into the water?' he would inquire, as he sat on a rock enjoying the afternoon sun. I would look closely to see the water rushing quickly downstream. My eyes would catch the glimpse of a fish, water beetles, flies touching the water, soaked wood floating along at the will of the water, rocks, and green plants.

"'I see the water,' I said. 'What else do you see?' he asked. 'Well, I see the fish,' I answered, because there were little minnows swimming around in the water. 'What else do you see?' he asked. 'I see the rocks,' I said. 'What else do you see?' he asked again. My eyes began to water a little as I stared intently, wanting so much to please my Grandfather by seeing everything he saw.

"'Ah, I see my reflection,' I responded proudly. 'That's good,' he replied confidently. 'What you see is your whole life ahead of you. Know that the Great One has a plan for you to be the keeper of everything you see with your eyes, 'cause every living thing is your brother and sister.' 'Even the rocks?' I questioned. 'Yes, even the rocks,' he answered, 'because they have elements of Mother Earth and Father Sky, just as we do.'

"'Remember to give thanks every day for all things that make up the Universe,' said my Grandfather. 'Always remember to walk the path of Good Medicine and see the good reflected in everything that occurs in life. Life is a lesson, and you must learn the lesson well to see your true reflection in the water'" (J. T. Garrett, cited in Garrett, 1996, p. 12).

## When Eagle Speaks

My father has shared so many powerful stories of his life experience with me, and I feel fortunate to be able to pass that along to my son. Maybe the spirit of the Eagle was whispering to my father that day when he sat by the river with his grandfather. His grandfather was considered a "spiritual man" and frequently didn't say a whole lot. That reminds me of a quote by the great Nez Perce leader, Chief Joseph, "It does not require many words to speak the truth" (Padilla, 1994, p. 45). To walk in step and beauty is to celebrate the deeper truths contained within the Sacred Dance of Life, to join the Circle with an open mind and an open heart, and to move at our own pace with clarity, kindness, joy, and a sense of calm. To walk in beauty is to understand and to practice the way of right relationship and to appreciate all of the beauty that exists both within and all around us and to help clients do the same.

Eagle asks, "Do you want to learn how to fly? Do you want to see great Creation through my eyes? Do you want to dance on the wind as I do?" When Eagle speaks, she speaks in the way that she moves. She speaks with her eyes, with her balance, with her presence. She speaks from the energy and power of the Four Directions, and their sacred flow. She speaks from the Galun'lati, the Sky World, from Alohi, Mother Earth, and from the center, ayeli, where the heart is born and reborn. She speaks from the truth that soars in her heart and in her spirit. And as she speaks, she walks in step and dances in beauty upon the wind.

## A Blessing Way

O Great One, I come before you in a humble manner, giving thanks for all things in Creation. I offer the clarity of my mind, body, spirit, and natural space in prayer to you, O Great One, for the spirit of all Creation. I offer great thanks and what gifts I have to the Four Sacred Directions and powers of the universe and I pray:

> To the spirit of Fire in the east,
> To the spirit of Earth in the south,
> To the spirit of Water in the west,
> To the spirit of Wind in the north.

I pray and give thanks to you, O Great One. I pray and give thanks to Mother Earth, Father Sky, Grandfather Sun, Grandmother Moon, and all our relations in the Greater Circle of Life. I thank you for your power, energy, and sacred gifts, because without you, I would not be able to live, and grow, and learn. I pray to you, giving thanks with the knowledge that everything is as it should be at any point in time. I ask that you help me see more clearly if I have ever harmed or hurt other living things. I pray to you, offering what gifts I have, that you may keep us, heal us, purify us, and protect us. I pray for all our relations that we may exist together in harmony and balance. "Sgi!"

## Summary and Conclusion

This chapter was presented to provide information on the Native way but also to help the reader step imaginatively into the Native world of the Circle. Within the Circle all of us are connected and our lives intertwined, life is sacred, and all around us are "relations"—Mother Earth, Father Sky, Eagle, Owl, and so forth. Counseling can help us to stay in "good relations" and live life to the fullest. This demands balance and effort to honor the connections *among* us, *between* us and the natural environment, and *between* us and the spirit world.

As counselors, we are privileged to help guide our clients on their own path to healing and balance. To do so requires courage, humility, and a willingness to experience life fully. Only then can we be wise and reliable guides.

### References

Aldred, L. (2000). Plastic shamans and astroturf sun dances. *American Indian Quarterly, 3,* 329–353.

Brendtro, L. K., Brokenleg, M., & Van Bockern, S. (1990). *Reclaiming youth at risk: Our hope for the future.* Bloomington, IN: National Education Service.

Deloria, V., Jr. (1994). *God is red: A Native view of religion.* Golden, CO: Fulcrum.

Dufrene, P. M. (1990). Exploring Native American symbolism. *Journal of Multicultural and Cross-Cultural Research in Art Education, 8,* 38–50.

Garrett, J. T., & Garrett, M. T. (2002). *The Cherokee full circle: A practical guide to ceremonies and traditions.* Rochester, VT: Bear & Company.

Garrett, J. T., & Garrett, M. T. (1996). *Medicine of the Cherokee: The way of right relationship.* Santa Fe, NM: Bear & Company.

Garrett, M. T. (2002). The four directions. In J. L. DeLucia-Waack, K. Bridbord, & J. S. Kleiner (Eds.), *Group work experts' favorite activities: A guide for choosing, planning, conducting, and processing* (pp. 119–122). Alexandria, VA: ASGW.

Garrett, M. T. (1999). Understanding the "Medicine" of Native American traditional values: An integrative review. *Counseling and Values, 43,* 84–98.

Garrett, M. T. (1998). *Walking on the wind: Cherokee teachings for harmony and balance.* Santa Fe, NM: Bear & Company.

Garrett, M. T. (1996). Reflection by the riverside: The traditional education of Native American children. *Journal of Humanistic Education and Development, 35,* 12–28.

Garrett, M. T., & Carroll, J. (2000). Mending the broken circle: Treatment and prevention of substance abuse among Native Americans. *Journal of Counseling and Development, 78,* 379–388.

Garrett, M. T., & Crutchfield, L. B. (1997). Moving full circle: A unity model of group work with children. *Journal for Specialists in Group Work, 22,* 175–188.

Garrett, M. T., & Garrett, J. T. (2002). Ayeli: Centering technique based on Cherokee spiritual traditions. *Counseling and Values, 46,* 149–158.

Garrett, M. T., & Garrett, J. T. (1997). Counseling Native American elders. *Directions in Rehabilitation Counseling: Therapeutic Strategies with the Older Adult, 3,* 3–18.

Garrett, M. T., Garrett, J. T., & Brotherton, D. (2001). Inner circle/outer circle: Native American group technique. *Journal for Specialists in Group Work, 26,* 17–30.

Garrett, M. T., & Myers, J. E. (1996). The rule of opposites: A paradigm for counseling Native Americans. *Journal of Multicultural Counseling and Development, 24,* 89–104.

Garrett, M. T., & Wilbur, M. P. (1999). Does the worm live in the ground? Reflections on Native American spirituality. *Journal of Multicultural Counseling and Development, 27,* 193–206.

Good Tracks, J. G. (1973). Native American non-interference. *Social Work, 17,* 30–34.

Hernandez-Avila, I. (2000). Meditations of the spirit: Native American religious traditions and the ethics of representation. *American Indian Quarterly, 20,* 329–353.

Herring, R. D. (1994). The clown or contrary figure as a counseling intervention strategy with Native American Indian clients. *Journal of Multicultural Counseling and Development, 22,* 153–164.

Hirschfelder, A., & Kreipe de Montano, M. (1993). *The Native American almanac: A portrait of Native America today.* New York: Macmillan.

Irwin, L. (1996). Themes in Native American spirituality. *American Indian Quarterly, 20,* 309–327.

Lake, M. G. (1991). *Native healer: Initiation into an ancient art.* Wheaton, IL: Quest Books.

Locust, C. (1988). Wounding the spirit: Discrimination and traditional American Indian belief systems. *Harvard Educational Review, 58,* 315–330.

Maples, M. F., Dupey, P., Torres-Rivera, E., Phan, L. T., Vereen, L., & Garrett, M. T. (2001). Ethnic diversity and the use of humor in counseling: Appropriate or inappropriate? *Journal of Counseling and Development, 79,* 53–60.

Matheson, L. (1996). Valuing spirituality among Native American populations. *Counseling and Values, 41,* 51–58.

Padilla, S. (1994). *A natural education: Native American ideas and thoughts.* Summertown, TN: Book Publishing Company.

Red Horse, J. G. (1997). Traditional American Indian family systems. *Families, Systems, & Health, 15,* 243–250.

Roberts-Wilbur, J., Wilbur, M., Garrett, M. T., & Yuhas, M. (2001). Talking circles: Listen or your tongue will make you deaf. *Journal for Specialists in Group Work, 26,* 368–384.

Russell, G. (1997). *American Indian facts of life: A profile of today's tribes and reservations.* Phoenix, AZ: Russell.

Spencer, P. U. (1990, Summer). A Native American worldview. *Noetic Sciences Review,* pp. 14–20.

Vick, R. D., Sr., Smith, L. M., & Iron Rope Herrera, C. (1998). The healing circle: An alternative path to alcoholism recovery. *Counseling and Values, 42,* 132–141.

Wilbur, M. P. (1999a). The rivers of a wounded heart. *Journal of Counseling and Development, 77,* 47–50.

Wilbur, M. P. (1999b). Finding balance in the winds. *Journal for Specialists in Group Work, 24,* 342–353.

# CHAPTER NINE

# Counseling Conservative Christian Couples: A Spiritually Sensitive Perspective

## Richard E. Watts

According to Miller, the mental health professions have developed to the point that many professionals are seeking to integrate rather than alienate the role of spirituality in human functioning. Evidence of this integrative quest

> is seen in a plethora of new books, in professional organizations, and in a more general resurgence of interest in religion and things spiritual, reflected even in the popular press. About 95% of Americans say that they believe in God. For many, spirituality and religion are important sources of strength and coping resources, and not infrequently people name them as the most important aspect of their lives, central to their meaning and identity. Many special populations cannot be understood at all without appreciating the history and centrality of religion in their community. It is a serious blind spot, then, not to understand or even ask about spirituality in our clients' lives.   (1999, p. xviii)

Historically speaking, most approaches to individual, couple, and family counseling have had either a neutral or negative position toward religion and spirituality. In recent years, however, many scholars and practitioners view spirituality as an important dimension to diversity, multiculturalism, and the therapeutic process, and they consequently urge counseling professionals to develop greater competency in treating clients from religiously and spiritually diverse backgrounds (Bishop, 1995; Burke & Miranti, 1995; Eriksen, Marston & Korte, 2002; Faiver, Ingersoll, O'Brien & McNally, 2001; Fukuyama & Sevig, 1999; Ingersoll, 1995; Kelly, 1995; Miller, 1999; Pate & Bondi, 1995; Richards & Bergin, 1997, 2000; Shafranske, 1996; Sperry, 2001; Walsh, 1999; Watts, 2000, 2001; Watts & Eriksen, in press; Wendell, 2003).

In fact, several authors have suggested that addressing religion and spirituality in couple and family counseling, my own specialty, is imperative and an essential aspect of clinical practice (Anderson, 1992; Burton, 1992; Doherty, 1999; Frame, 2000; Grizzle, 1992; Walsh, 1999; Wright, 1999). In my estimation, ignoring or discounting clients' spiritual perspectives and issues is both unethical and clinically inappropriate (Watts, 2000, 2001; Watts & Eriksen, in press). Thus, the importance of attending to clients' spiritual lives cannot be overemphasized.

## How I Developed an Interest in Spirituality and Counseling

The beginnings of my interest in spirituality and counseling may be traced to my seminary training where I studied, among other things, philosophy and world religions. During my last semester of seminary, I read *The Abolition of Man* by C. S. Lewis (1947). In this book, Lewis convincingly demonstrates the common moral and ethical foundation shared by major world religions and philosophies. This reading was transformative for me and gave me an appreciation of a variety of spiritual and philosophical perspectives.

Upon graduation from seminary, I began master's level counselor training and then entered doctoral work with an emphasis in marriage and family counseling. During my master's coursework, I began looking at the common ground between individual and systemic counseling theories and my perspective on spirituality. In addition, one of my professors included me in a research project examining the beliefs of counselors and clergy regarding the role of religious beliefs with a client struggling with depression (Holden, Watts & Brookshire, 1991). This research further whetted my appetite for investigating the interface of spiritual perspectives and counseling theory.

Early in my doctoral work I became attracted to the Adlerian approach to counseling. Two important reasons, among many, for this developing interest include the following: (1) the Adlerian perspective views spirituality in a positive light, and (2) I found substantial common ground between several strands of spiritual beliefs—including my own—and Adlerian psychology and counseling. Adlerian counseling's assumptions and characteristics readily facilitate work with culturally diverse clients, including religious and spiritual diversity. Furthermore, religious and spiritual issues are regularly addressed in the Adlerian literature (e.g., Ansbacher & Ansbacher, 1978; Arciniega & Newlon, 1999; Carlson, Watts & Maniacci, 2006; Dreikurs, 1971; Gold & Mansager, 2000; Hoffman, 1994; Jahn & Adler, 1933/1979; LaFountain & Mustaine, 1998; Manaster & Corsini, 1982; Mansager, 2000; Mosak & Dreikurs, 1967/2000; Mosak & Maniacci, 1999; Mozdzierz, 1998; Sweeney, 1998; Watts, 1999, 2000, 2003b; Watts & Eriksen, in press; Watts & Shulman, 2003).

## Using Spirituality in Counseling

### My Personal View of Spirituality

My personal view of spirituality is clearly theistic and relational. An ecumenical perspective similar to that which C. S. Lewis describes in his writings, my spirituality is rooted in teachings common to traditional Christianity regardless of denominational perspective and open to insights gleaned from other religious and spiritual perspectives. As Augustine (via Ambrose) affirmed, all truth is God's truth, wherever one may discover it.

Christian spirituality, as I understand it, is a relational spirituality. Biblical teachings are the primary anchor of meaning making in Christian spirituality, and the primary focus of the Bible is on relationships. The Bible affirms that humans have a three-fold relational responsibility— to God, to others, and to oneself—and most of the Bible addresses this three-fold responsibility (Elmore, 1986; Erickson, 1986; Grenz, 1994, 2001; Guthrie, 1981; Ladd, 1974). For example, the Ten Commandments (Exodus 20:1–17) are relationally focused. The first four address one's relationship to God (vv. 1–11). The following six address one's relationship to others (vv. 12–17).

Jesus' teachings powerfully confirm the strongly relational nature of Christian spirituality. When Jesus was asked to identify the greatest commandment in the Law, he stated, "You shall love God with all your heart, and with all your soul, and with all your mind. This is the greatest and foremost commandment. The second is like it: You shall love your neighbor as yourself. On these two commands depend the whole Law and the Prophets" (Matthew 22:37–40, New American Standard Bible). Therefore, spirituality, in my view, is about life lived in relationships: relationship with God and relationships with fellow human beings created in the image of God.

## Using Clients' Spirituality in Counseling: An Ethical Responsibility

Although I espouse a theistic and relational view of spirituality, I do not presuppose that clients must espouse my view of spirituality in order for me to be helpful. Various professional counseling ethical codes stress the need to respect clients' dignity, promote positive growth and development, and understand and respect cultural and religious/spiritual diversity (Frame, 2000). The clients' view of spirituality, as defined by the client, like their cultural values, must be respected and, if appropriate, included as a focal part of the counseling process (Watts, 2001). However, as Miller notes, "sensitivity and responsiveness to spiritual diversity do not require that one personally be a believer or share in clients' perspectives, any more than one must change skin color to respect and communicate across racial differences" (1999, p. xviii).

In my opinion, counselors who do not attend to religious and spirituality issues in counseling are practicing in a culturally insensitive and potentially unethical manner (Frame, 2000; Watts, 2001). That is, avoidance of these issues is not respectful of clients as persons, does not promote their growth and well-being, and is not respectful of their religious or spiritual diversity. Not attending to clients' religious or spiritual issues may risk a covert, even surreptitious, imposition of a counselor's values on the client. When counselors avoid these issues, clients may perceive or assume that their important spiritual values and beliefs do not matter and/or have no place in counseling (Watts, 2001). Thus, it is important for counselors to develop greater competency in religious and spiritual diversity so as to be as helpful as possible with spiritually diverse clients.

> It is through personal awareness and learning about diverse expressions of religion, spirituality, and the transpersonal that counselors can determine when it may be part of a presenting problem, and/or part of the solution. Multicultural counseling training provides an umbrella within which the religious, spiritual, and transpersonal may be considered. In addition, this area of inquiry overlaps with

ethics and values, and as such needs to be included in discussion of professional issues.     (Fukuyama, 2000, pp. 8–9)

## Using Clients' Spirituality in Counseling:
## A Clinical Perspective

Many clients may be hesitant or even afraid to see professional counselors because they are concerned that their religious or spiritual perspectives will be discounted, ignored, or even viewed as pathological (Bergin, Payne & Richards, 1996; Richards & Bergin, 1997, 2000). However, spirituality is a vital area for counselors to understand, because clients' spiritual beliefs typically provide the value system by which they view themselves, others, and the world. Without understanding their clients' spiritual perspectives, counselors are "operating with a vital value system and possibly even a member of the family, God, left at home and ignored" (Grizzle, 1992, p. 139). To ignore or discount clients' religious and/or spiritual issues in counseling is to close one's eyes to a crucial therapeutic factor. If clients perceive counselors as devaluing or ignoring the importance of their spirituality in the therapeutic process, they may become reluctant to share those beliefs or may terminate counseling. By neglecting to draw on clients' religious and spiritual values, "counselors lose the essence of the clients and deprive them of the opportunity to find meaning, strength, and support in their lives" (Benjamin & Looby, 1998, p. 98).

The question naturally arises, "what does one do if clients' spiritual beliefs are part of the problem?" There is a wealth of literature discussing how self-destructive beliefs and values can and should be challenged, while remaining more generally open to and using clients' perspectives on spirituality (e.g., Burke & Miranti, 1995; Burton, 1992; Jones & Butman, 1991; Kelly, 1995; Mansager, 2000; McMinn, 1996; Miller, 1999; Pargament, 1997; Propst, 1996; Richards & Bergin, 1997, 2000; Shafranske, 1996; Walsh, 1999; Warnock, 1989; Watts, 1992, 2000, 2001; Watts & Eriksen, in press; Watts & Trusty, 1997; Worthington, 1999). In addition, there are several established professional journals that address religious and spiritual issues in counseling and psychotherapy as a matter of course. Examples include *Counseling and Values,* the *Journal of Psychology and Christianity,* the *Journal of Psychology and Judaism,* the *Journal of Psychology and Theology,* and the *Journal of Transpersonal Psychology.* Furthermore, in recent years more general professional journals have had several issues or special sections, as well as occasional articles, dedicated to spirituality and counseling/therapy, for example, the *Family Therapy Networker* (Sept./Oct., 1990), *Journal of Family Psychotherapy* (2002, #1–4); and *Journal of Individual Psychology* (2000, #3).

## Adlerian Counseling as a Spiritually Sensitive Perspective: A Brief Overview*

As noted earlier, Adlerian counseling generally sees religion and spirituality in a positive light and works well with diverse religious and spiritual perspectives. The characteristics and assumptions of Adlerian theory are congruent with the cultural values of many minority racial and ethnic groups and affirm that the Adlerian counseling process is respectful of cultural diversity. Adlerian counseling goals are not aimed at deciding for clients what they should change about themselves (Arciniega & Newlon, 1999, p. 451):

> Rather, the practitioner works in collaboration with clients and their family networks. This theory offers a pragmatic approach that is flexible and uses a range of action-oriented techniques to explore personal problems within their sociocultural context. It has the flexibility to deal both with the individual and the family, making it appropriate for racial and ethnic groups.

These characteristics and assumptions of Adlerian counseling are equally important for working with spiritually diverse clients, as well.

### Adlerian Counseling: A Relational, Constructive Perspective

Adlerian counseling theory is a relational perspective (Carlson, Watts & Maniacci, 2006; Manaster & Corsini, 1982; Watts, 2003b). Humans are socially embedded and cannot be understood apart from their relational contexts. Adlerian theory considers both the socially embedded and relational nature of human knowledge and the personal agency of creative and self-reflective individuals within relationships. It embraces a holistic perspective that affirms that knowledge and experience are a

---

*Editor's Note: This contributor's integration of spiritual sensitivity with a particular approach to counseling (Adlerian) is offered as one possible model. The next several pages provide a succinct summary of Adlerian work and its overlap with spiritual themes. The case study that follows offers a rare glimpse into how such an integration is carried out in practice.

co-construction of self *and* others (Carlson, Watts & Maniacci, 2006; Watts, 2003b; Watts & Shulman, 2003). The cardinal tenet of Adlerian psychology, *Gemeinshaftsgefühl* (most commonly translated "social interest"), is obviously a social-contextual one. The word is also occasionally translated "community feeling." I believe both ideas (community feeling and social interest) are needed for a proper understanding of what Adler meant by *Gemeinshaftsgefühl;* that is, "community feeling" as the affective and motivational aspects of living and "social interest" as the cognitive and behavioral aspects.

Thus, true community feeling (that is, sense of belonging, empathy, caring, and acceptance for others) results in social interest (thoughts and behaviors that demonstrate caring for and contributing to the good of all humankind—"loving one's neighbor"—at both micro- and macro-systemic levels). Furthermore, true social interest is motivated by community feeling. This holistic conceptualization attends to cognitive, affective, and behavioral aspects of human functioning. Furthermore, Mosak (1995, p. 53) notes that *Gemeinshaftsgefühl* (or "social interest") is the Adlerian definition of mental health: "If we regard ourselves as fellow human beings with fellow feeling, we are socially contributive people interested in the common welfare, and by Adler's pragmatic definition of *normality,* mentally healthy."

Mosak (1995, p. 59) indicates as well that "Adler's psychology has a religious tone. His placement of social interest at the pinnacle of his value theory is in the tradition of those religions that stress people's responsibility for each other." He presents the Biblical mandate to love one's neighbor as oneself (Leviticus 19:18; Matthew 22:39; Mark 12:31; Luke 10:27) as a succinct illustration of Adler's concept of social interest. I have demonstrated elsewhere (Watts, 1992) that a strong parallel exists between Adler's social interest and the biblical Greek word *agape.* *Agape* is the highest form of love and is primarily volitional and self-giving rather than emotional and self-centered. *Agape,* like Adler's mature definition of social interest, exists as a possibility in every person and must be consciously developed in relationship with others. The famous "love chapter" in 1 Corinthians 13 provides an excellent strategic model of social interest based on biblical *agape.* Verses four through seven list fifteen attitudinal and behavioral descriptors of *agape* that resonate significantly with the descriptors of well-developed social interest discussed in the Adlerian literature. The shared characteristics of *agape* and social interest include, but are not limited to, perseverance, benevolence, humility, trustworthiness, altruism, unselfishness, and optimism (Watts, 1992). Both constructs—*agape* and social interest—ultimately address the mental health of individuals living in relational matrices. The person developing increased levels of *agape* or social interest is moving toward increased mental health. In the case of both constructs, however, *process* is the key word. In the course of this life, no one will ever reach absolute levels of *agape* or social interest.

Adlerian counseling is commonly viewed as consisting of four aspects or phases. The first aspect and, for most Adlerians, the most important, is entitled *relationship.* Because counseling occurs in a relational context, Adlerians focus on the development of a respectful, collaborative, and egalitarian counseling relationship with clients. Consistent with many religious and spiritual perspectives, Adlerian counseling emphasizes the importance of *encouragement.* Adlerian counseling considers encouragement to be a crucial aspect of human growth and development. Adler (1956) and Dreikurs (1967) believed that encouragement is essential for all relationships, counseling or otherwise. Stressing the importance of encouragement in counseling, Adler stated: "Altogether, in every step of the treatment, we must not deviate from the path of encouragement" (1956, p. 342). The process of encouragement includes demonstrating concern for clients through active listening and empathy; communicating respect for and confidence in clients; focusing on clients' strengths, assets, and resources; helping clients to generate perceptual alternatives for discouraging fictional beliefs and oppressive narratives; focusing on clients' efforts and progress; and helping clients see the humor in life experiences (Carlson, Watts & Maniacci, 2006; Watts, 2000, 2003b; Watts & Eriksen, in press; Watts & Shulman, 2003).

## Adlerian Counseling: An Integrative, Eclectic Perspective

Adlerian counselors are "technical eclectics," that is, they use a variety of cognitive, experiential, and behavioral techniques from various theoretical perspectives based on the unique needs and situation of each client (Manaster & Corsini, 1982; Mosak, 1995). Also, within the context of my understanding of Adlerian counseling, I often like to use procedures from postmodern approaches to counseling to engage clients in a spiritually reflective dialogue (Watts, 2003a, b; Watts & Eriksen, in press; Watts & Trusty, 2003; Watts & Shulman, 2003; West, Watts, Trepal, Wester & Lewis, 2001). By taking a "not knowing" position and allowing clients to be the "experts" regarding their spiritual beliefs and values, counselors may open space for clients to thoughtfully reflect upon the unique meanings they give their spirituality, both growth-enhancing and potentially growth-inhibiting meanings. Using reflective questions, counselors can also help clients explore additional or alternative possible meanings and behaviors *from within their framework of faith or spirituality.*

The idea of affirming clients' growth-promoting beliefs, and reinterpreting or challenging growth-inhibiting ones, is discussed extensively in literature across varying theoretical perspectives. Propst (1996, p. 394) states that modifying and transforming beliefs and assumptions resembles many aspects of spiritual expression. For example, Propst notes the similarity between cognitive restructuring and the religious idea of repentance, which means to "change one's mind about how one's self and the world is to be viewed." Thus, creating perceptual alternatives or cognitive restructuring could be described as "a type of spiritual transformation of the mind—a spiritual exercise" (1996, p. 394).

Counseling procedures and directives are often more acceptable to clients when described in a language in which they are comfortable. Creating a dialogue between their sacred writings or teachings (such as the Bible for Christians) and their discouraging beliefs and maladaptive behaviors may prove helpful. For example, when working with a devout Christian couple or family, a counselor may—when sufficient trust has been established—consider using Biblical passages in deconstructing and reconstructing clients' discouraging perspectives (Watts, 2000; Watts & Eriksen, in press).

Grizzle (1992, pp. 142–143) succinctly states that whereas counselors should be cautious in challenging the basic spiritual beliefs of clients

> it can be extremely helpful to point out in their own faith language how they may have followed one extreme principle to the exclusion of another within their own faith framework. Knowing these principles can help the practitioner address these belief systems in a faith supportive manner. . . . Often clients may have taken one aspect of belief to an extreme without recognizing the other balancing principle. By pointing this out within their faith framework, they may be able to modify their patterns without feeling their basic beliefs have been challenged.

The Bible is filled with stories of relationships and guidelines for living in relationship with others. "It deals with loneliness, discouragement, marriage problems, grief, parent-child relations, anger, fear, and a host of other counseling situations" (Collins, 1988, p. 22). The case study to follow demonstrates how a counselor may use these stories and guidelines for helping clients reflect upon or deconstruct current construals and then consider alternative interpretations.

## Case Study: "Why Are You Reading Her Mail?"

Gene and Marie (not their real names) were referred to me by their pastor. Members of a conservative Christian congregation, they both indicated that their Christian faith was foundational to them and that it was important for them to have a counselor who respected their beliefs and was comfortable working with them from a biblical perspective.

Gene was thirty-one and Marie twenty-five, and they had been married for almost three years. Gene and Marie met during his final year (of six) in the Army. Marie stated that she was first attracted to Gene because he was a "take charge" kind of person and she felt very safe because of Gene's "strong personality." Gene commented that he was attracted to Marie because she had strong Christian values and had no problem letting him "be the man in the relationship."

I asked the couple to tell me how they understood the problem that brought them to see me. They both conceptualized the situation in terms of their religious beliefs, albeit offering conflicting perspectives. I let both clients inform me about how they understood the relationship between their religious beliefs and their current marital strife. In summary, Marie complained that, although she agreed that "the husband should be the spiritual leader of the home," Gene was dictatorial and oppressive in his role as leader. She indicated that she began to experience discontent with his treatment of her near the end of their first year of marriage and had been struggling with depression for several months. Gene stated that Marie did not follow the Bible's mandate to submit to his leadership in the home. He suggested in session, as he had often suggested at home, that her feelings of depression resulted from her disobedience regarding the Bible's teaching of her role as a wife. Both Gene and Marie stated that they based their understanding of the roles of husband and wife on Ephesians 5:22–33.

In session two, we talked through their answers to the *How I Remember My Family Questionnaire* (Watts, 2000) and also created a genogram that included spirituality (Frame, 2000; Hodge, 2001). Both Gene and Marie remembered growing up in "chaotic" and "scary" homes where their fathers struggled with alcoholism and physically and verbally abused both the mothers and the children in the home. Gene's early memories centered on his need to be "in control" of his life, so that no one would treat him in an abusive manner again. Marie's early memories focused on finding someone to "rescue" her from an abusive situation.

The following transcription begins early in my third session with Gene and Marie. We began the session with each partner explaining their understanding of the Ephesians 5:22–23 passage and the intensity quickly escalated.

*Gene:* [In a loud voice] Well, whatever. The bottom line is that the Word of God clearly says that she [Marie] should respect me and submit to my leadership.

*Marie:* [In a somewhat resigned intonation] Yes, that's what it says. But that doesn't mean you get to be a dictator and treat me the way you do.

*Richard:* Okay, okay. Let's stop a second so I can get some things clear in my mind. First, it sounds like you both view the Bible as the Word of God and you both believe that your lives should match up with what it says. [They both nod.] And this passage in Ephesians is the basis for your understanding of the roles of husbands and wives in a Christian home. [Marie nodded, but Gene spoke.]

*Gene:* But she is not doing what it says! [Marie crossed her arms, sat back in her chair, lowered her head, and began to look at the floor.]

*Richard:* Before we get to that, let's take a look at that passage. [I reached over and picked up a Bible I brought to the session.] Are you both okay with my reading this passage from the New American Standard translation of the Bible? [They both agreed, and I read the passage below, Ephesians 5:22–33, out loud in session.]

> Wives, be subject to your own husbands, as to the Lord. For the husband is the head of the wife, as Christ is also head of the church, He Himself being the Savior of the body. But as the church is subject to Christ, so also the wives ought to be to their husbands in everything.     (vv. 22–24, New American Standard Bible)

*Gene:* See, there it is; that's what I'm talking about!

*Richard:* Please, let me finish the passage before we talk about it. [Gene nodded and sat back with his arms crossed.]

> Husbands, love your wives, just as Christ also loved the church and gave Himself up for her; that He might sanctify her, having cleansed her by the washing of water with the word, that He might present to Himself the church in all her glory, having no spot or wrinkle or any such thing; but that she should be holy and blameless. So husbands ought to also to love their wives as their own bodies. He who loves his own wife loves himself; for no one

ever hated his own flesh, but nourishes and cherishes it, just as
Christ also does the Church, because we are members of His body.
For this cause a man shall leave his father and mother, and shall
cleave to his wife; and the two shall become one flesh. This mystery is great; but I am speaking with reference to Christ and the
church. Nevertheless let each individual among you also love his
own wife even as himself; and let the wife see to it that she respect
her husband.    (vv. 25–33, New American Standard Bible)

**Richard:**    Well, Gene, you're right; it does say that the wife should be
subject to and respect her husband.

**Gene:**    That's what I've been trying to tell you. And she is not following what the Word of God teaches.

**Richard:**    Well, I'm frankly a bit confused after reading this passage.

**Gene:**    How so? It seems very clear to me.

**Richard:**    Well, the part of this passage you've been talking about,
who is it addressed to?

**Gene:**    What do you mean? It is the Word of God, it is addressed to
everyone.

**Richard:**    It's addressed to husbands or wives?

**Gene:**    Oh, okay. Well, it's addressed to wives.

**Richard:**    So it seems that you have been reading mail addressed to
Marie.

**Gene:**    Well, even so, it still says what it says; that she should submit
to my leadership.

**Richard:**    True enough. And we can look at that with Marie after we
read the mail addressed to you.

**Commentary:**    We then revisited the lengthy part of the passage addressed specifically to husbands that begins with "Husbands, love your
wives," and I asked both partners to provide "summary" words regarding
how husbands should love their wives. Gene begrudgingly participated.
The list that we co-constructed included *unselfish, sacrificial, nourishing,
cherishing,* and *as himself.*

**Richard:**    Gene and Marie, where do you—each individually—think
the Bible gives the clearest description for how love "behaves"?

**Gene:**    [almost impulsively responding and smiling] Well, I thought
for sure you would know that. It is 1 Corinthians 13.

*Marie:*    I agree. In fact, we had that passage in our wedding.

*Richard:*    So, that's the passage you both think best describes how love "behaves." Do you mind if we look at it together? [They both nodded affirmatively, and I turned to 1 Corinthians 13:4–8a and read it out loud.]

> Love is patient, love is kind, and is not jealous; love does not brag and is not arrogant, does not act unbecomingly; it does not seek its own, is not provoked, does not take in account a wrong suffered, does not rejoice in unrighteousness, but rejoices with the truth; bears all things, believes all things, hopes all things, endures all things. Love never fails.    (1 Corinthians 13:4–8a, New American Standard Bible).

The passage in Ephesians says, "Husbands, love your wives," and earlier we constructed a list based on the part of the passage addressed to the husband. How similar does it look to the part of 1 Corinthians 13 we just read?

*Gene:*    Yeah, it looks somewhat similar.

*Marie:*    I think it has very similar ideas; it just uses different words.

*Richard:*    It seems to me that these two passages together give a pretty good picture of how the Bible says that husbands should love their wives.

*Gene:*    [in a raised voice] Yeah, okay. But when are you going to talk about what the wife should do?

*Richard:*    That's a good question, Gene. You want to know when we will talk about you being the leader of the home and how Marie is to follow your leadership.

*Gene:*    Right.

*Richard:*    [looking to Marie] When Gene, as the spiritual leader of the home, is setting the example by genuinely trying to follow the Bible's teachings on how a husband should love his wife, do you think you, Marie, will be ready to talk about how you are to follow the Bible's teachings on respecting his leadership?

*Marie:*    Sure.

**Commentary:**    My guess at this juncture was that Marie's withdrawal and depression were an attempted solution to Gene's controlling and oppressive behavior. Gene, however, responded by becoming even more controlling rather than less. Both partners were simply increasing the intensity of behavior that was not working rather than trying something different. Based on some previous success with couples sharing similar religious views, I decided to engage the couple in a dialogue with another passage from the Bible (1 Cor. 13:4–8) that might add additional meaning to the Ephesians 5:22–23 passage and might help them reflect upon their present understandings and open space for considering alternative interpretations. As noted earlier in this chapter, the passage from 1 Corinthians 13 resonates with the Adlerian understanding of mental health and healthy relational behavior.

My initial focus was to engage Gene because I sensed he had the most power in the relationship. By having him consider the Ephesians 5:22–23 passage in conjunction with 1 Corinthians 13:4–8, I hoped to put him in a state of dialogical dissonance. That is, either he had to deny that he believed the Bible was the Word of God and was authoritative for *his* life (which I was fairly certain he would *not* do), or he would have to consider beginning to treat Marie as the Bible states husbands should love their wives. I was much less concerned about Marie's following the biblical mandate for wives. She had earlier implied that if she felt loved instead of intimidated, she would like for Gene to be the spiritual leader of the home, and responded affirmatively when I explicitly asked her about it.

Although he remained polite for the remaining few minutes of this session, I could tell Gene was frustrated and angry. I tried to reflect my sense of his feelings, but Gene denied he was angry. I was concerned about Gene pursuing a third option: dropping out of counseling all together.

My intuition was accurate. Marie called the day before the next session to say that Gene did not like me and the way I did counseling. She indicated that Gene had instead scheduled an appointment to talk with their pastor. Two days later Marie called to say that the meeting with the pastor had not gone well. She indicated that their pastor had essentially agreed with me that Gene's oppressive behavior was inappropriate. Marie stated that Gene was considering visiting a different church.

I did not hear from either Marie or Gene for over two months. To my surprise, however, I received a phone call from Gene nine weeks after our last appointment. Marie had previously scheduled all the appointments, but Gene scheduled this one. Frankly, the thought of him coming in the room and punching me crossed my mind. When Gene and Marie arrived, I was further taken aback by what Gene said as we began the session. He apologized. He went on to say that over the two month period he continually struggled with what we discussed in our last session.

*Gene:*   It seems everywhere I went and everyone I listened to, in one way or another, talked about how a husband should treat his wife. I was listening to [James] Dobson on the radio and he was talking about how husbands should love their wives. We visited a different church and the pastor was doing a series on marriage. That Sunday he did a sermon on "Husbands love your wives." After that, I actually did not go to church for two weeks because of the inner struggle I was going through. The second of the Sundays that I stayed home, I watched a Christian speaker on TV, and sure enough, part of his sermon addressed how good family relationships start with husbands loving their wives. I could not get away from what we had talked about. And it started seeming pretty obvious to me that God was trying to tell me something. So I quit praying for God to straighten out Marie and began praying about what I should do. Well, I went and apologized to my pastor and talked with him about my experience. He suggested that Marie and I resume counseling. I went home and talked with Marie about it, and then I called you.

**Commentary:**   Often when we are immersed in a difficult situation, we selectively attend only to the problem and ignore alternative perspectives that might lead to useful solutions. When we are able to step out or step away from difficulties and reflect on the situation, however, new and preferred meanings often emerge. This transformative process appears to be true from both counseling and spiritual points of view, and I believe this happened in Gene and Marie's case. In the over-two-month period after our previous session, Gene encountered a number of experiences that supported the work initiated in our counseling sessions and further helped open him to considering a new relational reality. During this period, Marie chose to be supportive rather than withdrawing. In addition, she chose not to push Gene but gave him space and support through his struggle. Gene's decision to call for an appointment and Marie's decision to neither push nor pull away from Gene seemed to me indicative of a new openness on both their parts.

*Richard:*   I'm really glad you decided to continue with counseling. Sounds like you are at a better place to begin working to improve your relationship.

*Gene:*   Yeah, but here's the deal for me. I don't know what to do or how to do it. I feel out of control right now. My parents had a lousy marriage and I've never been very good with relationships beyond kind of a surface level. And I've always structured my life so I can be in charge and in control. I don't know what else to do; it's all I know. Where do I . . . [hesitating] . . . Where do *we* [putting his hand on Marie's] start?

*Richard:*  This has been a very meaningful time and I'm impressed with how you've handled it. Gene, I think the fact that you are here and are willing to work on the relationship is a great start. In our time together, you two can help each other discover and begin developing the kind of relationship you both want. Does that sound like something you're both willing to do?

*Gene:*  Yes.

*Marie:*  Absolutely. I want our marriage to work.

## Concluding Case Commentary and Follow-Up

We reviewed the contents of our previous sessions. I shared with Gene and Marie that, although the Bible passages discussed in earlier sessions provide general guidelines, it seems to me that they do not specifically delineate how each couple would embody the various characteristics of a loving relationship—one manifesting increasing levels of *agape* and social interest. In other words, within the general guidelines of a loving relationship, each couple must construct and work out their own unique way of being together.

We spent the remainder of the session helping them generate meanings of a loving relationship, specific to their unique relationship but consistent with their faith perspective. The passage from 1 Corinthians 13 largely informed our dialogue. Prior to the next session, I asked them to keep a journal and jot down some answers to the following reflective questions:

- If you were acting "as if" you were the couple you would like to be, what would you be doing differently? And what would your relationship look like?

- If a close friend were to see you six months from now and you had made significant progress toward the loving relationship you want, how would that person say you were acting differently as a couple?

During the next session, we talked through their journal reflections and co-constructed a list of "as if" behaviors indicative of how they will act as a couple as they move toward the relationship they desire. After constructing the list, I helped both partners rank the "as if" behaviors in terms of difficulty (from "least" to "most"). Their homework prior to the next session was for each partner to focus on one or two of the "least" difficult behaviors from the list they created. It was my hope that beginning with the least difficult behaviors would increase the likelihood of success, and increase Gene and Marie's perceived relational self-efficacy.

During the following session, we discussed the behaviors that were focused on for the week. Both indicated that, although there was some initial difficulty, they began to sense a difference in their relationship. Both felt more hopeful because it seemed that their partner was trying to make a difference. We discussed what they appreciated about each partner's behaviors, how the behavior helped the relationship, and how each partner might expand the behaviors for their partner's benefit. We talked about the relationship between each partner's behavior and how both saw it as congruent with the biblical passages discussed earlier. Near the end of the session, each partner selected two additional behaviors for the coming week to add to the previously selected ones.

This pattern continued for the remaining seven sessions. Frankly, some behaviors were more easily integrated into the relationship than others were. As the tasks increased in perceived difficulty, Gene or Marie (or both) occasionally resorted to prior dysfunctional patterns. We processed these situations during sessions and discussed perceptual and behavioral alternatives. In addition, we worked on communication and conflict management skills, and intimacy exercises and rituals. Gene and Marie decided to begin adding only one behavior between sessions, and some of these required further discussion, evaluation, and adjustment. However, they demonstrated significant progress because their relationship developed to the point where they could discuss, evaluate, and adjust without the escalating hostility that was evident when they first presented for counseling.

Over the next eighteen months, either Gene or Marie would occasionally call and set up a follow-up or "booster" session with the partner's permission. Gene called it a "tune-up" and we would typically address newly emerging issues in their relationship.

## Concluding Thoughts

The goal of this chapter was to help counselors develop a greater level of comfort and competency in working with conservative Christian clients; in this case, a couple. Spirituality is a vital area for counselors to understand because clients' spiritual beliefs are often crucial for understanding clients' self and relational perspectives.

Counselors choosing to ignore or discount religious or spiritual issues in clinical settings may actually impose their values on clients because clients may assume that their important spiritual values and beliefs do not matter or have no place in counseling. Regardless of whether counselors share the religious or spiritual perspectives of their clients, they can demonstrate respect for and interest in clients' spirituality, develop greater competency with the spiritually diverse populations with whom they work, and thereby use the potential strengths and assets contained within their clients' spirituality to facilitate growth and development.

## Select Recommended Resources for Spiritually Sensitive Counseling

(*) indicates resources especially useful for working with conservative Christian clients

*Clinton, T., & Ohlschlager, G. (2002). *Competent Christian counseling* (vol. 1). Colorado Springs: WaterBrook/Random House.

*Fall, K. A., Holden, J. M., & Marquis, A. (2004). Integral counseling: The prepersonal, personal, and transpersonal in self, culture, and nature. In *Theoretical models of counseling and psychotherapy* (pp. 419–479). New York: Brunner-Routledge.

*Grizzle, A. F. (1992). Family therapy with the faithful: Christians as clients. In L. A. Burton (Ed.), *Religion and the family: When God helps* (pp. 139–162). New York: Haworth Pastoral Press.

Hinterkopf, E. (1998). *Integrating spirituality in counseling: A manual for the experiential focusing method*. Alexandria, VA: American Counseling Association.

*Jones, S. L., & Butman, R. E. (1991). *Modern psychotherapies: A comprehensive Christian appraisal*. Downers Grove, IL: InterVarsity Press.

Mansager, E. (Guest Editor). (2000). Holism, wellness, spirituality [Special Issue]. *Journal of Individual Psychology, 56*(3).

Miller, G. (2003). *Incorporating spirituality in counseling and psychotherapy: Theory and technique*. Hoboken, NJ: Wiley.

Miller, W. R. (Ed.). (1999). *Integrating spirituality into treatment: Resources for practitioners*. Washington, DC: American Psychological Association.

Nielsen, S. L., Johnson, W. B., & Ellis, A. (2001). *Counseling and psychotherapy with religious persons: A rational emotive behavior therapy approach*. Mahwah, NJ: Lawrence Erhlbaum.

Richards, P. S., & Bergin, A. E. (1997). *A spiritual strategy for counseling and psychotherapy*. Washington, DC: American Psychological Association.

Sperry, L. (2001). *Spirituality in clinical practice: Incorporating the spiritual dimension in psychotherapy and counseling*. Philadelphia: Brunner-Routledge.

Walsh, F. (Ed.). (1999). *Spiritual resources in family therapy*. New York: Guilford.

Watts, R. E. (2001). Addressing spirituality issues in secular counseling and psychotherapy. *Counseling and Values, 45,* 207–217.

*Worthington, E. L. (Ed.). (1993). *Psychotherapy and religious values.* Grand Rapids, MI: Baker.

## References

Adler, A. (1956). Encouragement. In H. L. Ansbacher & R. R. Ansbacher (Eds.), *The individual psychology of Alfred Adler* (pp. 341–342). New York: Norton.

Anderson, D. A. (1992). Spirituality and systems therapy: Partners in clinical practice. In L. A. Burton (Ed.), *Religion and the family: When God helps* (pp. 87–101). New York: Haworth Pastoral Press.

Ansbacher, H. L., & Ansbacher, R. R. (Eds.). (1978). *Cooperation between the sexes: Writings on women, love, and marriage.* New York: Norton.

Arciniega, G. M., & Newlon, B. J. (1999). Counseling and psychotherapy: Multicultural considerations. In D. Capuzzi & D. F. Gross (Eds.), *Counseling & psychotherapy: Theories and interventions* (2nd ed., pp. 435–458). Upper Saddle River, NJ: Merrill/Prentice Hall.

Benjamin, P., & Looby, J. (1998). Defining the nature of spirituality in the context of Maslow's and Rogers' theories. *Counseling and Values, 42,* 92–100.

Bergin, A. E., Payne, I. R., & Richards, P. S. (1996). Values in psychotherapy. In E. P. Shafranske (Ed.), *Religion and the clinical practice of psychology* (pp. 297–326). Washington, DC: American Psychological Association.

Bishop, D. R. (1995). Religious values as cross-cultural issues in counseling. In M. T. Burke & J. G. Miranti (Eds.), *Counseling: The spiritual dimension* (pp. 59–72). Alexandria, VA: American Counseling Association.

*Burke, M. T., & Miranti, J. G. (Eds.). (1995). *Counseling: The spiritual dimension.* Alexandria, VA: American Counseling Association.

Burton, L. A. (Ed.). (1992). *Religion and the family: When God helps.* New York: Haworth Pastoral Press.

Carlson, J., Watts, R. E., & Maniacci, M. (2006). *Adlerian therapy: Theory and practice.* Washington, DC: American Psychological Association.

Collins, G. R. (1988). *Christian counseling: A comprehensive guide* (rev. ed.). Dallas: Word.

Doherty, W. J. (1999). Morality and spirituality in therapy. In F. Walsh (Ed.), *Spiritual resources in family therapy* (pp. 179–192). New York: Guilford.

Dreikurs, R. (1971). *Social equality: The challenge for today.* Chicago: Adler School of Professional Psychology.

Dreikurs, R. (1967). *Psychodynamics, psychotherapy, and counseling.* Chicago: Alfred Adler Institute of Chicago.

Elmore, V. O. (1986). *Man as God's creation.* Nashville, TN: Broadman.

Erickson, M. J. (1986). *Christian theology.* Grand Rapids, MI: Baker.

Eriksen, K., Marston, G., & Korte, T. (2002). Working with God: Managing conservative Christian beliefs that may interfere with counseling. *Counseling and Values, 47,* 48–68.

Faiver, C., Ingersoll, R. E., O'Brien, E., & McNally, C. (2001). *Explorations in counseling and spirituality: Philosophical, practical, and personal reflections.* Belmont, CA: Brooks/Cole-Wadsworth/Thomson Learning.

Frame, M. W. (2000). Spiritual and religious issues in counseling: Ethical considerations. *The Family Journal: Counseling and Therapy for Couples and Families, 8,* 72–74.

Fukuyama, M. A. (2000, Spring). Integrating spirituality into marriage and family counseling. *The Family Digest, 12*(4), 1, 7–9.

Fukuyama, M. A., & Sevig, T. D. (1999). *Integrating spirituality into multicultural counseling.* Thousand Oaks, CA: Sage.

Gold, L., & Mansager, E. (2000). Spirituality: Life task or life process? *Journal of Individual Psychology, 56,* 266–276.

Grenz, S. J. (2001). *The social God and the relational self.* Louisville, KY: Westminster John Knox.

Grenz, S. J. (1994). *Theology for the community of God.* Nashville, TN: Broadman & Holman.

Grizzle, A. F. (1992). Family therapy with the faithful: Christians as clients. In L. A. Burton (Ed.), *Religion and the family: When God helps* (pp. 139–162). New York: Haworth Pastoral Press.

Guthrie, D. (1981). *New Testament theology.* Downers Grove, IL: InterVarsity Press.

Hoffman, E. (1994). *The drive for self: Alfred Adler and the founding of Individual Psychology.* Reading, MA: Addison-Wesley.

Holden, J. M., Watts, R. E., & Brookshire, W. (1991). Beliefs of professional counselors and clergy about depressive religious ideation. *Counseling and Values, 35,* 93–103.

Ingersoll, R. E. (1995). Spirituality, religion, and counseling: Dimensions and relationships. In M. T. Burke & J. G. Miranti (Eds.), *Counseling: The spiritual dimension* (pp. 5–18). Alexandria, VA: American Counseling Association.

Jahn, E., & Adler, A. (1979). Religion and individual psychology. In A. Adler (1979), *Superiority and social interest* [Edited by H. L. Ansbacher & R. R. Ansbacher] (pp. 271–308). New York: Norton (original work published in 1933).

Jones, S. L., & Butman, R. E. (1991). *Modern psychotherapies: A comprehensive Christian appraisal.* Downers Grove, IL: InterVarsity Press.

Kelly, E. W. (1995). *Spirituality and religion in counseling and psychotherapy: Diversity in theory and practice.* Alexandria, VA: American Counseling Association.

Ladd, G. E. (1974). *A theology of the New Testament.* Grand Rapids, MI: Eerdmans.

LaFountain, R. M., & Mustaine, B. L. (1998). Infusing Adlerian theory into an introductory marriage and family course. *The Family Journal, 6,* 189–199.

Lewis, C. S. (1947). *The abolition of man.* New York: Macmillan.

Manaster, G. J., & Corsini, R. J. (1982). *Individual Psychology.* Itasca, IL: Peacock.

Mansager, E. (Guest Editor). (2000). Holism, wellness, spirituality [Special Issue]. *Journal of Individual Psychology, 56*(3).

McMinn, M. R. (1996). *Psychology, theology, and spirituality in Christian counseling.* Wheaton, IL: Tyndale.

Miller, W. R. (Ed.). (1999). *Integrating spirituality into treatment: Resources for practitioners.* Washington, DC: American Psychological Association.

Mosak, H. H. (1995). Adlerian psychotherapy. In R. J. Corsini & D. Wedding (Eds.), *Current psychotherapies* (5th ed., pp. 51–94). Itasca, IL: Peacock.

Mosak, H., & Dreikurs, R. (2000). Spirituality: The fifth life task. *Journal of Individual Psychology, 56,* 257–265 (original work published in 1967).

Mosak, H. H., & Maniacci, M. (1999). *A primer of Adlerian psychology: The analytic-behavioral-cognitive psychology of Alfred Adler.* Philadelphia: Accelerated Development/Taylor & Francis.

Mozdzierz, G. J. (1998). Culture, tradition, transition, and the future. *Journal of Individual Psychology, 54,* 275–277.

*New American Standard Bible.* (1977). La Habra, CA: Lockman Foundation.

Pargament, K. I. (1997). *The psychology of religion and coping.* New York: Guilford.

Pate, R. H., & Bondi, A. M. (1995). Religious beliefs and practice: An integral aspect of multicultural awareness. In M. T. Burke & J. G. Miranti (Eds.), *Counseling: The spiritual dimension* (pp. 169–176). Alexandria, VA: American Counseling Association.

Propst, L. R. (1996). Cognitive-behavioral therapy and the religious person. In E. P. Shafranske (Ed.), *Religion and the clinical practice of psychology* (pp. 391–408). Washington, DC: American Psychological Association.

Richards, P. S., & Bergin, A. E. (1997). *A spiritual strategy for counseling and psychotherapy.* Washington, DC: American Psychological Association.

Richards, P. S., & Bergin, A. E. (Eds.). (2000). *Handbook of psychotherapy and religious diversity.* Washington, DC: American Psychological Association.

Shafranske, E. P. (Ed.). (1996). *Religion and the clinical practice of psychology.* Washington, DC: American Psychological Association.

Sperry, L. (2001). *Spirituality in clinical practice: Incorporating the spiritual dimension in psychotherapy and counseling.* Philadelphia: Brunner-Routledge.

Sweeney, T. J. (1998). *Adlerian counseling: A practitioner's approach* (4th ed.). Muncie, IN: Accelerated Development.

Walsh, F. (Ed.). (1999). *Spiritual resources in family therapy.* New York: Guilford.

Warnock, S. D. M. (1989). Rational-emotive therapy and the Christian client. *Journal of Rational-Emotive and Cognitive Behavior Therapy, 7,* 263–274.

Watts, R. E. (2003a). Reflecting "as if": An integrative process in couples counseling. *The Family Journal: Counseling and Therapy for Couples and Families, 11,* 73–75.

Watts, R. E. (2003b). Adlerian therapy as a relational constructivist approach. *The Family Journal: Counseling and Therapy for Couples and Families, 11,* 139–147.

Watts, R. E. (2001). Addressing spirituality issues in secular counseling and psychotherapy. *Counseling and Values, 45,* 207–217.

Watts, R. E. (2000). Biblically-based Christian spirituality and Adlerian therapy. *Journal of Individual Psychology, 56,* 316–328.

Watts, R. E. (1999). The vision of Adler. In R. E. Watts & J. Carlson (Eds.), *Interventions and strategies in counseling and psychotherapy* (pp. 1–13). Philadelphia: Accelerated Development/Taylor & Francis.

Watts, R. E. (1992). Biblical agape as a model of social interest. *Individual Psychology, 48*, 35–40.

*Watts, R. E., & Eriksen, K. (in press). Counseling conservative Christian clients: An integrative Adlerian perspective. In D. Sandhu (Ed.), *Spirituality as a fifth force*. Alexandria, VA: American Counseling Association.

Watts, R. E., & Shulman, B. H. (2003). Integrating Adlerian and constructive psychotherapies: An Adlerian perspective. In R. E. Watts (Ed.), *Adlerian, cognitive and constructivist theories of counseling and psychotherapy: An integrative dialogue* (pp. 9–37). New York: Springer Publishing Company.

Watts, R. E., & Trusty, J. (2003). Using imaginary team members in reflecting "as if. " *Journal of Constructivist Psychology, 16*, 335–340.

Watts, R. E., & Trusty, J. (1997). Chaos and Christianity: A response to Butz and a Biblical alternative. *Counseling and Values, 41*, 88–96.

Wendell, R. (2003). Lived religion and family therapy: What does spirituality have to do with it? *Family Process, 42*, 165–179.

West, J. D., Watts, R. E., Trepal, H. C., Wester, K. L., & Lewis, T. F. (2001). Opening space for client reflection: A postmodern consideration. *The Family Journal: Counseling and Therapy for Couples and Families, 9*, 431–437.

Worthington, E. L., Jr. (1999). *Hope-focused marriage counseling: A guide to brief therapy*. Downers Grove, IL: InterVarsity Press.

Wright, L. M. (1999). Spirituality, suffering, and beliefs: The soul of healing with families. In F. Walsh (Ed.), *Spiritual resources in family therapy* (pp. 61–75). New York: Guilford.

# Nurturing the Spirituality of Our Youth

## Mary Alice Bruce

Behold, a sad commentary by Jim, age fourteen:
"I couldn't get my teachers to take my questions and ideas seriously. I thought this was what school was going to be about. There was such a big deal about going off to first grade, but I kept waiting for us to talk about life—you know, why we're all here, what this world's about. The nature of the universe. Things like that. When I'd ask or say my ideas just to sort of get things going, there would be dead silence, and then the teacher would move on to spelling or something. I thought, *okay, I guess we're getting the basic stuff this year, and then we'll get into the good stuff in second grade. I can wait that long if I have to.* Well, second grade came and went, and it wasn't any better—maybe worse—since we didn't even get to play as much. By fourth grade I remember thinking, *I must be an alien. These people don't understand. I'm not a social zero: I have friends. But no one, especially not the teachers, are talking about this. School seems not to be very interested in my questions or any questions really; it is all about the answers. We're only supposed to give them the right answer*" (Hart, 2004, p. 45).

In my work as a school counselor, I often saw children eagerly arrive in kindergarten with lots of questions and then leave our schools punctuated as periods rather than as exclamation points for life. As in the story above, our youth are ready to be part of something larger than themselves, such as humanism and spirituality, and yet their spiritual awareness and needs are often unrecognized. Increasingly, evidence has emerged regarding powerful spiritual experiences of children (Hart, 2004).

Children's spiritual evolution appears to be sequenced, somewhat parallel to cognitive and psychosocial development. This process involves finding a purpose, connectedness, and meaning in life while offering hope and strength (Ingersoll & Bauer, 2004). The major spiritual models of development include that of Genia (1990) whose five-stage faith development model through the lifespan expands concepts of object relations theory and psychoanalytic development psychology. Fowler's six-stage model of faith development suggests that the genuine human experience brings forward a universal quality of meaning making throughout life. Meanwhile, Chandler, Holden, and Kolander (1992) conceptualized a model of spiritual wellness that consists of six major dimensions: intellectual, emotional, physical, social, occupational, and spiritual. They believed that regaining and maintaining spiritual balance throughout various life events can help a person progress to higher levels of development. Wilber (1995) offered the Integral model with progressions of spirituality that bring together mind, body, soul, and spirit through stages of human and systems development. Valuable insights, practices, and ideas are offered by these models that may offer guidance in nurturing spirituality.

Benner (1989) described spirituality as a sense of interconnectedness and oneness, the heartfelt desire to find self-identity, meaning, and a place in the world. Building on Benner's description, I define spirituality as a quest for transcendence beyond the limits of the self to a higher level of meaning that leads to authenticity, connectedness, compassion, and oneness in and with the Universe. The steps leading to transcendence are awareness and self-knowing, which are hard to achieve in our stressful world of hurry-up materialism, alienation from each other, and push-button gratification. Because one consequence of nontranscendence is restless dissatisfaction, I believe our youth are yearning for an identity of harmony in truth by seeking a higher power and the nurturance of their spirituality.

When surrounded by the conflict and chaos of the world, everyday life can involve a variety of challenges for our youth, ranging from peer pressure and drugs to their own internal struggles with anger and loneliness. As such, our children often doubt themselves, as well as the adults in their world. Spiritual nurturance may offer hope and strength in order to cope with the difficulties and stressors that seem to surround them (Elkins & Cavendish, 2004). Without spiritual care and the accompanying comfort it provides, the ability for kindness, compassion, and empathy may diminish, replaced by discontent and anger. As Victor Frankl stated, "Men are most apt to kill when they feel overcome by meaninglessness" (1984, p. 179). How can we nurture youth to know themselves and develop values, positively connect with others, feel unity with a higher power, and find meaning in life?

## A Personal Sense of Spirituality

As a young child, I remember my basic awareness of the differences between right and wrong. I appreciated that our family routines of attending weekly Sunday school and church services, as well as midweek youth activities, provided a firm anchor for my life. However, throughout those years, I also remember lots of whispered negative conversations about breaking away from the structure and demands of our families. As my self-awareness grew and conscience developed, I started to realize the rewards but also the expectations, limits, and consequences of society. As such, I noticed myself increasingly making moral decisions in the context of my midwestern culture, family beliefs, and religious practices—decisions that led to the development of a strong sense of compassion and altruism.

My adolescent years yielded a sense of belonging and connection to a community of empathic adults who helped me along my journey. Consistent and realistic limits set by my parents, plus caring adults at school and church, helped me make many wise choices. During frequent meetings at our house and elsewhere, those adults greeted my siblings and me with warmth and care. Now, I reflect with pleasure about my dual-career parents and their various community service activities. On the whole, I enjoyed affirmations and was blessedly nurtured.

Because of my increased self-awareness, I began to watch myself more closely as I interacted with friends and classmates. I observed how I talked with others and what I did with others. I considered and wondered how and/or if I was being myself, truly congruent with me or not. Where was my center, my balance point, the real me? I was trying to discover myself, to learn about myself, to know myself.

According to Duff (2003), after awareness comes self-knowing as the foundation for spiritual growth. To move forward with self-knowing on the path of spiritual development, one must examine one's thoughts, become aware of motivation underlying thoughts, judge thoughts as helpful or harmful, and learn how to control one's thoughts in a positive manner, continuing to observe and learn what is not known about one's self.

Soon, I began to question my own purpose in life. I wondered so often, *Why am I here?* As I stumbled and grew in awareness, acceptance, and self-understanding, I realized that I was quite busy with doing instead of being. I wanted to quiet down and be still. I needed to find a way, the way for me. Then, I worked to step aside and step back from those thoughts, detach from my thoughts so as to transcend them into unity or oneness. Meditation was a useful tool that provided me a means to focus or concentrate on nothing in order to open up into something bigger. Simple self-soothing also gave me practice in calming myself into peace and tranquility that could lead deeper into myself and then beyond in order to know myself from moment to moment. In summary, I believe that spiritual development encompasses awareness, self-knowing, and then transcendence (Duff, 2003). I still struggle on my journey.

## Spiritual Development as Part of a School Counseling Program

Because of my work as coordinator of our university school counseling program and associate professor of counselor education, and prior to that as a mathematics teacher and school counselor, I believe that we can nurture the spiritual growth of P–12 students while meeting the legitimate educational requirements of those students. Spirituality is "integral to an education for meaning, social justice, character, depth, and wisdom" (Hart, 2004, p. 39).

Emotion is the core of consciousness and brings forward spiritual aspects of life (Scheindlin, 2003). However, in the United States we currently face challenges in integrating the affective and cognitive domains in our schools due to the intense emphasis on knowledge acquisition and the accountability demands of federal legislation such as the No Child Left Behind Act of 2001 (U.S. Department of Education, 2005). Even Goleman (1995), widely known for his research regarding emotional intelligence, based his work on business professionals who are successful in the achievement-oriented Western business world where priority is given to managing and controlling emotions rather than expressing and experiencing them. Furthermore, according to Scheindlin (2003), the "emotional intelligence movement" in the schools may simply feed into the rational, logical, suppression of emotional richness needed to enhance the spiritual dimensions of our youth. In order to reduce violence and maintain order and discipline in the school environment, this new "movement" focuses on controlling emotions through rationality rather than connecting with them and developing emotional richness. While valuable in helping children to manage difficult emotions, this focus may have the unintended side-effect of hindering students from fully experiencing positive emotions (such as love or compassion) that can lead to the experience and exploration of one's spirituality. The contemporary school counselor needs to be comfortable with managing AND experiencing the full range of emotions and feelings, while having strategies at hand for providing opportunities to develop both feelings and students' spirituality.

Unlike Great Britain which now requires the moral and spiritual development of children to be taught by means of the curriculum in the schools (Bottery, 2002), public schools in the United States are very clear regarding the legal separation of church and state. However, I believe that while keeping the required distance from religion, we can provide natural conditions and opportunities for spiritual development and nurturance in public schools.

Based upon the American School Counseling Association's (ASCA) National Standards for School Counseling Programs (Campbell & Dahir, 1997) that focus on academic, personal/social, and career development, professional school counselors can consult and collaborate with teachers to offer a rationale and to create conditions that are opportune for students' emotional experiences and thus spiritual growth by means of the necessary steps of awareness and self-knowing that lead to transcendence (Duff, 2003). Already, counselors, teachers, and other adults respond daily to the behaviors and ways of students, since after all we are not emotionally neutral in our interactions. By means of our attitudes, beliefs, and values, we establish the emotional culture of the school while acknowledging values of the surrounding community and society.

In the everyday life of the school, a secondary school counselor can collaborate with teachers to broaden student emotional experiences that lead to self-awareness and self-knowing while simultaneously achieving state content standards as well as ASCA standards during normal classroom times. Collaborative teaching offers such an experience for students when the social studies teacher and counselor present case scenarios about conflicts, and then consider together with the students strategies to manage conflicts as well as articulate the accompanying emotions and resulting self-awareness. An elementary school counselor can also easily bring opportunities for spiritual development via affective and cognitive domains into classroom guidance and small-group work. For example, Duff (2003) suggested several practical, non-therapeutic teaching and learning strategies that are helpful in creating conditions that are opportune for spiritual development as well as academic achievement.

During the awareness stage as the first step of spiritual development, counselors can intentionally disclose how they feel and what is happening for them in everyday life, and then encourage students to express their own thoughts and emotions, thereby increasing their awareness of self and others. Students must be helped to learn the language of feelings and then share with others. Adults in the school can model and thus give students the license to fully express themselves in genuine ways. Youth can be taught to keep an open mind, noticing, realizing, and respecting their internal voice and external influences.

The next step in creating awareness is the encouragement of children to observe themselves and each other and how they are in the world. How do they interact with other people, examine ideas, and think? Students can study how they themselves are motivated and how the world tries to affect them. Students can reflect, discuss with peers and adults, and thus learn appropriate emotional responses associated with good mental health. Counselors can wonder aloud to students, "Are your self-observations in keeping with your dream for life, for your life as you choose it, as you notice your way of behaving, thinking, feeling, and overall being in the world with others?" (Bruce & Cockreham, 2004).

Self-knowing is another component of spiritual development (Duff, 2003). Learning about self, realizing patterns of thought, understanding origins of thoughts, beginning to take control of one's thoughts, and being in the moment are some of the ways of increasing self-knowing. Stepping back into one's self can lead to the very center that offers self-knowing. To nurture self-knowing, counselors can have students make a list of facts about themselves, such as their strengths relative to specific career ideas. As students write their lists, counselors can help students notice what comes to mind, how others respond and react to their lists, and what then emerges for them as they relate to each other.

Another strategy for enhancing self-knowing is to have students notice their thoughts and then consider the thoughts that seem useful and those that seem harmful. For example, during math, a student may comment, "I never can get any of these problems right." In response, the teacher or counselor may wonder, "Where did that come from? Who says 'never' to you?" Students may then begin to realize how and from where their negative thoughts develop. As students observe, reflect, and articulate their thoughts, they learn about themselves, understand themselves better, and then begin to be able to decide how to positively support themselves moment to moment.

The next step of spiritual development is transcendence, which Duff (2003, p. 233) described as "a state that goes beyond the normal feeling of living." In transcendence, I believe that a person steps out of the attachments of the world and truly experiences what is inherent in being, giving way to the truth of one's self, a connection with energy and oneness. One of the best procedures for the development of transcendence is meditation, a process that can also help develop strategies for effective learning. A counselor collaboratively working with a social studies teacher regarding conflict management may say to the students, "Wow, lively discussion, lots of thoughtful comments about using an avoidance strategy in managing conflicts. Let's take a moment here to quiet ourselves, a few minutes of concentrated peace before we switch to a different strategy. Relax, close your eyes, if you choose; quiet your thoughts, and soon I'll start us up again with your fresh eyes."

A counselor can also help students move in the direction of transcendence with exercises in concentration, which can then merge into nothingness. Take time to focus on one object; perhaps the students can focus on the shape of a trapezoid during a geometry lesson as a step into nothingness. "Let's take two minutes to really focus on this object. Allow yourself to step into real concentration. Go for that focus without thinking." And then afterwards, "How was that to step into the zoom focus, into nothingness? Now you may feel even more energized to learn with an open mind!"

## Case Study of a Friendship Group

In the middle school where I was a counselor, the eight members of this Friendship Group were selected because of teacher and parent referrals relative to the overall purpose of the group, which was to facilitate psychosocial growth, with specific goals of increasing self-awareness, improving communication skills, and enhancing interpersonal relationships. According to Ingersoll and Bauer (2004), such a purposeful psychosocial environment nurtures spiritual wellness and growth. Letters sent home to parents and caretakers told of the Friendship Group opportunity that was offered to their children. In the letters, I presented the group's purpose and goals and made the curriculum easily available for parental review.

We met during a rotating study block time for forty-five minutes a week for the second quarter of the academic year. The group included seventh and eighth graders with four boys and four girls whose socioeconomic status, or SES, ranged from the low income of a single parent to parents providing very comfortable support. The ages of the group

members were from twelve to fourteen years; the ethnicities represented
were Latino and European-American, and their academic achievement
ranged from average to high (see Table 10.1).

## Creating Awareness

I begin this section on awareness with the third session of our group. As
the school counselor, I was familiar with these students because I knew
and enjoyed them through their activities as elementary students or in
this middle school. My intent with these group members was to continue to enhance emotional awareness, expression, and responses in an
appropriate and respectful manner so as to create awareness of their authentic selves (Bruce & Cockreham, 2004).

I welcome you, the reader, to join us today as the students enter the
counseling office. They sit in chairs at the round table after choosing a
squish ball or modeling clay to keep their hands busy. For myself, I
choose a note pad and pencil for doodling while we talk. As with most
school counselors, I have lots of interesting items such as magnets,
games, paper, and markers as well as little stuffed animals to help focus
the excess physical energy of middle school students.

Jen offers her usual bright smile and greeting as she enters with Kelli,
a very personable eighth grader. Leslie and Suzie arrive moaning after an
algebra test. Meanwhile, John and Carl come in laughing together as
they reflect about yesterday's football practice.

*Jen:*  I am so glad to be here today.

*Brian* (a boy already taller than anyone else in eighth grade):   Well,
it's not such a good day for me.

*Mary Alice:*  So, what is going on with everyone? How are you feeling
and doing? Brian, start us off—sounds as if you are ready.

*Brian:*  My folks are on me right and left. Be careful about this,
be careful about that. Did you get that assignment done? Where is
the trust?

*Carl:*  Bummer, geez, I know how they can be.

*Mary Alice:*  Hmmmm, sounds like Carl gets the picture. Help us all
understand, Brian.

*Brian:*  Last night, it was all about the term paper due in social studies
at the end of the quarter. Had I started the outline? Was I getting
material? They are on my case.

*Mary Alice:*  All of that sort of triggered frustration or ???

TABLE 10.1   Group Members

| Name | Age | Description |
|------|-----|-------------|
| Leslie | 12 | White female, high achievement, high SES |
| John | 13 | White male, high achievement, low SES |
| Carl | 14 | Hispanic male, high achievement, average SES |
| Bill | 13 | White male, average achievement, average SES |
| Jen | 12 | White female, average achievement, average SES |
| Brian | 14 | White male, low achievement, high SES |
| Kelli | 14 | White female, average achievement, average SES |
| Suzie | 13 | White female, high achievement, low SES |

*Brian:*   Yea, and then I got mad, just went to my room to get away.

*Leslie:*   I get tired of my parents with all that kind of stuff too. Just always making sure that we look good.

*Bill:*   And sometimes all that drives me crazy.

*Mary Alice:*   Impressive that you realize and talk about what goes on inside of you. How about others? What goes on inside for you as you notice these external forces?

The group members continue to articulate some of the emotions that come up for them in everyday life, especially as a result of interactions with adults.

*Mary Alice:*   It is normal to have some challenges that we handle all by ourselves or discuss with our friends. Good for you all that you are so aware of what goes on inside you, what you are thinking in your head and feeling in your heart. And kudos for talking about it, that's a sign of maturity! And now, as you notice what you do and how you feel, how does that fit with you as a person?

*Suzie:*   Sometimes, I am sort of ashamed that I get so mad.

*Carl:*   Yeah, me too. I just have to do like Brian, get away from it.

*Kelli:*   I used to scream, and then my parents would scream at me, plus ground me and everything. Sometimes I used the silent treatment. Guess I am going to try getting away somewhere, then come back to talk.

*John:*   I think that's why football helps. I can get away with my friends, and I'm in action.

*Bill:*  I just go to the computer. At home, I just get to those video games and I can calm myself so I can go back and deal with it. My parents know that I need time alone, and then we can talk. It's like I made this switch from elementary school, I can decide and know what to do, instead of just kicking stuff.

Bill's insight sets off more discussion about how the members are becoming aware of themselves. The more they talk, the more they realize that they are growing and learning. They almost visibly puff up with knowing themselves.

*Mary Alice:*  So many insightful comments about yourselves today, good going! Communication and relationship skills are looking good, and we know that there will be setbacks sometimes too. We just keep learning about ourselves and how to be better. Well, our time is up, so goodbye; I'll think about you this week.

## Self-Knowing

As the weeks pass, we continue the focus on authentic communication, improving connections with others, and taking steps into self-knowing. With this stage of the process leading to transcendence, I create conditions that support students to discover and understand themselves as they are in the moment. Being present in the moment and intending to understand moment by moment can help them discover, appreciate, and use their unique selves (Duff, 2003; Bruce & Cockreham, 2004).

*Mary Alice:*  Welcome, welcome, before you sit down, choose a pen or marker and a piece or two of colored paper for yourself. Sit anywhere around the room. You are going to work alone, and then we'll get around the table and see what everyone has done.

*Jen:*  Great, something different, so relaxing here. Come sit by me, Leslie.

*Carl:*  Oh, good, can we draw?

*Mary Alice:*  Yes, if you choose. First, take a moment to just be yourself. Put aside everything around you. Let's be quiet for a moment or two.

It takes a couple minutes for everyone to settle and calm themselves. I sit on the floor with my eyes closed, until we realize a minute or so of consistent silence.

*Mary Alice:*    Please think about yourself ten years from now. You have started a new job; you are on your career path. Let us know your strengths for this career. Use your paper to draw, list, or somehow be ready to show us and talk with us about your strengths. Help us know you better. OK everyone? OK, let's go.

So as to join the activity and connect, I draw too. I will share if time permits. To honor the students' need to focus, I do not roam around during this activity.

*Mary Alice:*    Does anyone need more time before we come together at the table? Okay, a couple more minutes and I'll check again . . . everyone ready? Great, come on over. Who wants to start us?

*Suzie:*    You all know that I am good at math, even if I'm not great at drawing, and that will help me be a professor. Here's my picture of me dreaming about algebra, and my mind is just clicking away. See the sparks of energy in the air. I work at lightning speed.

*John:*    And that's just how you are Suzie. You are so smart in math. You've always been fast doing your math work.

*Leslie:*    Yes, and that's why it's fun to sit by you in algebra, 'cause you work hard and like it. I like it too.

*Mary Alice:*    Suzie, how is it to notice things about yourself and then hear from your friends?

*Suzie:*    I feel proud, and I guess I never thought about working hard. It doesn't seem like hard work. It's more like a game that I play using all my brain power. Hmmm, I do play hard.

*Mary Alice:*    Congrats first for noticing and knowing about you, plus congratulations for listening to your friends think aloud about you and how you learn.

*Suzie:*    Thanks, everyone.

*John:*    Well, I'll go next. You all can see here that I am tackling someone on the field during a game. I am good at football, and I'm good at working on a team. So all that helps me plan for a pro football career or coaching or being a leader on a business team and then coaching on the weekends.

*Carl:*    Yep, you get along with everybody, but you are way tough as a linebacker. Kind of two sides to you.

*Jen:*    I agree, Carl. I remember that you stopped to help us when we were trying to get the car wash set up for Spanish Club that day.

All those buckets, coupling the hoses and everything, and you're not even in the Spanish Club.

*Kelli:* Lots of football players, not you two (indicating John and Carl), act cool with themselves, ignoring everybody else. So we get mad. But you both usually talk with everyone. You both are good at being friendly but also aggressive on the football field.

*Mary Alice:* I see a lot of heads nodding in agreement with what's being said. Hmmm, what's going on inside you this very moment, John?

*John:* I'm surprised. I just didn't understand that me being me and helping other people was something that special. I like working together with other people. Thanks everyone.

One by one, the students show their papers and explain their strengths and what they found out about themselves. As described above for Suzie and John, other members comment, and then I check in with the student before we move on to the next member. I work hard to pace us so as to offer all members a chance to share their strengths and receive comments from others during this too brief session. In closing, I set the stage for the next group session.

*Mary Alice:* Thanks to everyone for sharing some of your heart today. I admire how well you know yourselves. Between now and the next session, please notice what you think and say and do, and whether that is what you really want to think, say, and/or do, and whether that noticing might lead to increased awareness of yourself and others.

In the following weeks, we will explore some of the hurtful statements that others say to us or say about us behind our backs or hurtful statements that we say about ourselves. Also, we will identify other painful experiences and try to find ways to respond that promote an understanding of who we really are, behind some of our masks (Bruce & Cockreham, 2004). As we become more authentic and know more about ourselves, we can live more in the present, not on cruise control (Tolle, 1999).

As I talk with the group members, I facilitate their stretching to realize that there is a higher level of meaning beyond each of us, and to move toward the spiritual dimension of self-knowing that inherently underlies our communication and relationship skills.

## Transcendence

Creating a peaceful, calming space and going beyond one's self to a universal oneness is yet another spiritual dimension. I frame this as an opportunity to help the group members ease away from anxiety and the resultant stress of a hectic, pressure-packed school day. Activities that incorporate focus, concentration, and self-soothing are appropriate and logical for stress reduction, energy renewal for more effective teaching and learning, as well as spiritual development.

*Mary Alice:*    Great to see you all this week. Come in and find a comfortable spot, maybe at the table, a chair, or on the floor, wherever. We will try something soothing today. I know that as the end of the quarter approaches, we may fall into a stress trap every now and then. This exercise helps get you out of those traps and can give you a freer mind and more energy. Is everyone willing and ready to try this?

*Leslie:*    I'm ready to experiment with getting out of a stress trap!

*Jen:*    Me too

*Bill:*    Me three, ha!

*Mary Alice:*    Love that humor. Okay, great. I call this the Quiet Focus. Start letting your eyes wander around the room and choose an object on which you want to focus. When you have found something, just let your eyes settle on it. And then, mentally step back into yourself. Let your eyes rest on the object while you quiet and calm yourself. It's okay to close your eyes if you wish, and see the object in your mind. Sometimes our minds try to talk to us during this, so just put away the thoughts and quietly focus. Let yourself settle; step back into yourself, and see yourself as calm. I'll be silent for some minutes as we do this Quiet Focus.

The students are silent, moving a bit and adjusting themselves for comfort. Several make quick eye contact with each other, but then they settle and begin. I allow five solid minutes for this initial session. And then . . .

*Mary Alice:*    Well, everyone. How are you?

*Kelli:*    Calmer, hard to stop thinking though.

*Mary Alice:*    How did you help yourself?

*Kelli:*    Just kept removing the thoughts and looking at the wooden turtle there.

*Jen:*   Yeah, looking at something helps me, I think.

*Suzie:*   I really had to look at something boring so as to keep my mind from wondering about it. I started looking at the clock and realized that it moved and it reminded me of my time crunch. I switched and focused on the chair leg.

*Mary Alice:*   Insightful, thank you all. And others?

*Bill:*   I kept thinking of all the things I have to do too. Plus, I could feel my heart beating and hear my stomach growling, so it was hard.

*Carl:*   Maybe if we had some music.

*Mary Alice:*   Yes, I agree, this is hard. This is about staying aware and being with yourself in the now. Practice is very helpful. We can try some music. Is everyone up for having another try right now? Fine, we'll add music and notice how everyone is.

Moving into transcendence is a challenge. Facilitating students' control of their mind chatter and self-soothing is a helpful start. Next, I ask students to switch from the Quiet Focus and surge as if to mentally open themselves to the entire world and universe, being one with all that is. One tip that previous students have shared for this step is to achieve the Quiet Focus and then widen or open their eyes letting the energy surge through them as they open up to the void of everything. With a feel of freedom and clarity, the students are more than ready to be themselves in the world.

## Concluding Thoughts

In the United States, public schools offer much knowledge to students that may be considered external information, while opportunities for spiritual development call for nurturance of the knowing that comes from within, an inner life of awareness and self-knowing. Youth must be given the freedom and support to pursue both kinds of knowledge in order to balance traditional educational demands and spiritual nurturance.

Teaching spirituality is not the purpose; rather, nourishing our youth's full potential is the goal. As demonstrated, counselors and other adults can appropriately incorporate strategies that enhance effective learning, address youth's innate spiritual dimension, and provide opportunities for spiritual development. Fast-paced knowledge acquisition must be balanced with time for reflection, meaning, and transcendence.

## References

Benner, D. G. (1989). Toward a psychology of spirituality: Implications for personality and psychotherapy. *Journal of Psychology and Christianity, 8,* 19–30.

Bottery, M. (2002). Globalization, spirituality and the management of education. *International Journal of Children's Spirituality, 7,* 131–143.

Bruce, M. A., & Cockreham, D. (2004). Enhancing the spiritual development of adolescent girls. *Professional School Counseling, 2,* 334–342.

Campbell, C.A., & Dahir, C.A. (1997). *Sharing the vision: The national standards for school counseling programs.* Alexandria, VA: American School Counselor Association.

Chandler, C. K., Holden, J. M., & Kolander, C. A. (1992). Counseling for spiritual wellness: Theory and practice. *Journal of Counseling & Development, 7,* 168–175.

Duff, L. (2003). Spiritual development and education: A contemplative view. *International Journal of Children's Spirituality, 8*(3), 227–237.

Elkins, M., & Cavendish, R. (2004). Developing a plan for pediatric spiritual care. *Holistic Nursing Practice, 18*(4), 179–184.

Fowler, J. W. (1991). Stages in faith development. *New Directions for Child Development, 52,* 27–45.

Frankl, V. E. (1984). *Man's search for meaning.* New York: Washington Square Press.

Genia, V. (1990). Interreligious encounter group: A psychospiritual experience for faith development. *Counseling and Values, 35,* 39–51.

Goleman, D. (1995). *Emotional intelligence.* New York: Bantam Books.

Hart, T. (2004). The mystical child: Glimpsing the spiritual world of children. *ENCOUNTER: Education for Meaning and Social Justice, 17*(2), 38–49.

Hay, D. with Nye, R. (1998). *The spirit of the child.* Grand Rapids, MI: Zondervan Press.

Ingersoll, R. E., & Bauer, A. (2004). An integral approach to spiritual wellness in school counseling settings. *Professional School Counseling, 7,* 301–308.

Scheindlin, L. (2003). Emotional perception and spiritual development. *International Journal of Children's Spirituality, 8*(2), 179–193.

Tolle, E. (1999). *The power of now: A guide to spiritual enlightenment.* Novato, CA: New World Library.

United States Department of Education (2005). *Stronger accountability.* Retrieved April 22, 2005 from *www.ed.gov/nclb/accountability/index.html.*

Wilber, K. (1995). *Sex, ecology, spirituality: The spirit of evolution.* Boston: Shambhala.

❧

# CHAPTER ELEVEN

# Incorporating Spirituality into Rehabilitation Counseling and Coping with Disability

## Henry McCarthy

Interest in spirituality has burgeoned over the past two decades. This is evidenced by increased appearance and appreciation of publications on the topic in both academic circles and popular culture, including several special issues of scholarly journals (e.g., Hafferty, 1995; Thoresen, 1999; Vash, 2001) and cover stories in national news magazines. Some observers (e.g., Gregory, 1994; Larson, Wood & Larson, 1993) have described this interest as a paradigm shift. The continuing discussion and debate have made spirituality a more popular but no less controversial topic. The research question that has probably received the most attention is certainly germane to this chapter; that is, the wellness benefits of being spiritual or religious. The reader is referred to comprehensive state-of-the-art evaluations of this topic (e.g., Hill & Pargament, 2003; Miller & Thoreson, 2003). Other reviews have focused on the research exploring connections between religion/spirituality and both global measures of health (Powell, Shahabi & Thoreson, 2003) and mediating physiological processes such as immune function (Seeman, Dubin & Seeman, 2003).

## Dimensions of Spirituality

Personally, I view spirituality in three dimensions, as a resource for (a) understanding our existence, (b) balancing the demands of daily living, and

(c) actualizing one's self. Roughly speaking, one might label these the philosophical, sociological, and psychological dimensions of spirituality. Each of these dimensions will be described in turn and then coordinated with common concerns expressed by persons with a disability. Relevant characteristics of the counseling process will also be described.

## Understanding the Mystery of Existence

Spirituality calls to mind a variety of terms: Higher Power, Supreme Being, soul, supernatural, consciousness, cosmos, Divine Order, inter-connectedness, flow of energy, metaphysical, mystical, transcendence, transpersonal, Truth, unity. Constructs such as these demonstrate that spirituality offers us a domain of ideas and images about the creation, meaning, and eventualities of Life that can be incorporated as given or personalized by the individual. This dimension of spirituality is derived from elements of various world religions and schools of philosophy, although it cannot be reduced to the tenets of any single religious or philosophical system. The function of this aspect of spirituality is to shape each individual's evolving schema for grappling with the "big questions" of life, to facilitate the pursuit of wisdom that helps people to fathom cosmic existence and their place in it. As Pargament noted: "Much of classic religious literature takes the form of a dialogue between the divine and a seeker of meaning, the perplexed individual who wonders why there is evil, pain, and inequity in the world and how one should live amidst so much confusion" (1997, p. 48). The commonality of such spiritual questioning is supported by Levine's (1999) contention that children and adults of varying cognitive capacity and cultural sophistication nonetheless demonstrate comparable (even "isomorphic") experiences of spirituality.

## Balancing the Demands of Overloaded Lifestyles

Since the re-emergence of spirituality as a New Age marvel, much discussion in the literature and popular press has centered around distinguishing it from the concept of religion. Miller and Thoreson (2003) capsulated the distinction thus: "the field of religion is to spirituality as the field of medicine is to health" (p. 28). At times, it is helpful or important to distinguish between religion and spirituality. Many desire to do so because religion, despite its professed intentions, has a sad history of being a source of embittered divisiveness. As Deepak Chopra noted, "We have squeezed God into the volume of a body and the span of a lifetime; given God a male identity, an ethnic background; made him a tribal chief and gone to war" (Sachs, 2005, p. 10). Also, the distinction between religion and spirituality can be beneficial to maintain in situations that would raise concerns about overstepping the bounds of separation of church and state, a boundary that is ingrained as well as conflicted in our national consciousness (McCarthy, 1995). I have often found it more useful to distinguish how spiritual values differ from those of contemporary technocratic culture (see Table 11.1). Current lifestyles in technologically advanced societies, especially the United States, tend to become desiccated by non-nurturing expectations or obsessions rooted in excessive materialism (e.g., Kanner & Kasser, 2003), competition, and individualism (e.g., Putnam, 2000). Spiritual perspectives and practices can save us from overindulgence or desperation by providing an oasis from the mundane minutiae and depleting burdens of our high-tech, low-touch contemporary culture (McCarthy, 1999; Moore, 1992). Expressions of such spiritually redeeming values and rejuvenating rituals include holy ground, sacred space, sanctuary, compassion, blessed community, acceptance, contemplation, meditation, gratitude, healing, sacrifice, service, serenity, silence, simplicity, prayer, altruism, conscience, forgiveness, justice. Among these, the phenomenon of forgiveness and its therapeutic impact have drawn recent attention in the counseling literature (e.g., Baskin & Enright, 2004).

### Actualizing the Self

Spirituality can also serve as a guide and support to optimize the resources, choices, challenges, and transitions in our lives. This aspect of spirituality was cogently capsulated by that master of theory and research on self-actualization, Abraham Maslow: "The human being needs a framework of values, a philosophy of life, a religion or religion surrogate to live by and understand by in about the same sense that he needs sunlight, calcium or love" (1968, p. 206). Terms and processes indicative of this dimension of spirituality include authenticity, awakening, life path, life journey, life lesson, hope, meaning, destiny, mission, vocation, reflection, belief, integrity, vision, transformation, grace, wisdom, spirit guide, stewardship, surrender. Seeing the human developmental lifespan in universal themes and challenges, Vash identified commonalities among "human growth or psychological development or rehabilitation or whatever you prefer to call it" (1981, p. 130). She also argued for applying spiritual frameworks to understand and shape not just the traditionally inspiring but also the strange or discomforting manifestations of the struggle toward self-actualization:

> Would some mental disorders cause less pain and suffering, even disappear, if society would change its mind and respond differently

TABLE 11.1    Comparison of Technocratic Priorities and Spiritual Values

| Technocratic Priorities | Spiritual Values |
| --- | --- |
| expertise and planning | intuition and vision |
| reductionistic specialization | holistic integration |
| control and productivity | being in harmony |
| focus on the future | living in the moment |
| external selection | internal choice |
| legal accountability | self-responsibility |
| rugged individualism | creation of community |
| achieved status | inborn sacredness |
| material ownership | resource stewardship |
| competition and conquest | acceptance and embracing |
| eradicating disease | illness as a lesson and path |
| power, speed, strength | peace, balance, wellness |

to people whose atypical behavior now earns them clinical labels? . . . [C]linicians involved in the Spiritual Emergence Network report that patients with characteristics indistinguishable from symptoms of mental illness progress to levels of functioning higher than their pre-onset levels following treatment regimens that exclude medication and instead offer guidance for spiritual journeys. The Spiritual Emergence Network is based on the contention that many so-called mental illnesses are, in fact, emergent spiritual crises among people with extraordinarily high potential for self-actualization.   (Vash, 1994, p. 8)

## Relevance of Spiritual Dimensions to Counseling and Disability-Related Issues

We all yearn for understanding when faced with existential questions, solace when overburdened by daily living, and guidance when taking a step toward self-actualization. In addition to the usual existential, lifestyle, or self-actualization needs that bring people to seek fulfillment in spirituality, dealing with a disability can often create other reasons that may stimulate such a search. Nosek and Hughes (2001, pp. 22–23) have convincingly explained the

undeniable yet sadly ignored unity between spirituality and rehabilitation. Both are journeys of discovery. Both are paths toward defining who you are, how you relate to your universe, and where you are headed. This process of definition is punctuated by points of change, a convergence of readiness for a new awareness and an event that provides the momentum. For many people, disability is one such point of change.

In particular, the intrusion of a traumatic disability jolts one from an "auto-pilot" existence, giving one not only pause but usually an altered body and sometimes a brush with death en route. Understandably, any of these traumatic events can prompt pondering of "the most fundamental questions in the mind and heart of the person with a new disability, such as 'Why me?' 'Is this God's will?' 'Why doesn't God heal me?' and 'Did I do something to deserve this?'" (Mitchell, 2002, pp. 52–53). In arguing for an existential approach to counseling within rehabilitation, Beck elaborated its construct of "encouragement" and suggested that "the counselor could work on reducing the fear of spiritual nothingness and finding the purpose that gives the person's life meaning" (1999, p. 337).

If it does nothing else, even moderate disability magnifies one's vulnerability to daily stress. Consider the following concomitants of disability for many persons: extra energy and time requirements to perform self-care regimens; decreased opportunities for achievement because of architectural and attitudinal barriers; and reduced resources due to wage loss from unemployment or underemployment, expenses for treatment or equipment, and isolation from networks of social support. Many spiritually evolved persons who are handicapped by these forces believe that ongoing acceptance of disability can itself constitute a spiritual practice. For example, Bruno explained: "The goal of Buddhism is to treat each and every moment as a meditation, without craving, clinging or 'shoulding,' to be completely and fully present in the here and now. Imagine turning all the things you hate doing, that are hard and take so long to do because of physical limitations, into meditations—bathing, dressing, even your bowel program!" (1999, p. 37).

Functional deficits are not the only, nor are they even the major, source of frustration for most persons with a disability. The bumper sticker, "Your attitude is my biggest handicap," drives home that viewpoint. Wright (1983, 1988) has extrapolated a variety of general principles of human information processing to specific problems in the perception of disability as a social stimulus. Her point was to show how discrimination against persons with disabilities is not simply a matter of blatant prejudice or negative stereotypes, but is a more "fundamental negative bias" that needs to be guarded against to avoid unintentional underestimation, overprotection, or disempowerment of clients or loved ones with a disability. One such unwitting perceptual tendency is the "spread effect" (Wright, 1983), whereby a single salient deficit (such as an obvious speech disability) can get easily generalized by the observer to skill areas (such as cognitive and emotional functioning) that are actually unaffected, but are perceived or anticipated to be similarly limited. This results in additional stressors associated with lowered social valuation of, and societal investment in, the disabled person as a whole. If individuals with a disability then internalize these messages, the negative psychological impact can become compounded by diminished self-esteem.

Self-actualization and personal development are potentially complicated by disability. For example, experiences in formative career exploration can be constrained by inaccessible school and work environments, and unaccommodating gatekeepers. Indeed, the purpose of rehabilitation as a profession is to maximize the potential and participation of people with disabilities by developing compensatory strategies for circumventing the personal limitations and societal barriers that create the handicaps they experience.

Within the disability studies literature, Carolyn Vash has been the most innovative proponent for developing a psychospiritual perspective for understanding and utilizing experiences of adversity across the lifespan. She proposed her own Maslow-like hierarchy of adjustment, ultimately allowing for "transcendence" of the disability:

*Level I: Recognition of the Facts.* Disability is seen as a tragedy and has negative valence.

*Level II: Acceptance of the Implications.* Disability is seen as an inconvenience that can be mastered and has neutral valence.

*Level III: Embracing of the Experience.* There is appreciation of the fact that the disability has been, is, and will continue to be a growth catalyst if allowed to be so. Disability, like all other life experiences, is seen as an opportunity or gift and has positive valence.

> Naturally, there is a period of time before reaching Level I when the person fails to acknowledge even the facts; and acknowledgment and denial alternate in and below consciousness throughout life for most disabled people. (Vash & Crewe, 2004, pp. 150–151)

Additional publications (Vash, 1995, 2003) amplify her self-actualization theory by taking a narrative approach to exploring the spiritual dimensions of her own disability identity and career development.

### Rationales for Counselor Competence and Comfort with Spirituality

Many aspects of spirituality are consonant with values that shape counseling, rehabilitation, and other helping professions. In an introductory counseling textbook, Morgan (2000, p. 176) lists five aspects (numbers added): "Attention to the spiritual dimension of a person leads to (1) an attitude of respect for the whole person, (2) a valuing of his or her beliefs and meaning making, (3) a visioning of the counseling room as a sacred space in which life stories are told, (4) authentic encounter is encouraged, and (5) change—even transformation—is facilitated." Clients' right to receive care that respects their individual spiritual values was recently added to the standards set by the Joint Commission on Accreditation of Healthcare Organizations (Nowitz, 2005).

From its origins, the field of rehabilitation has been attuned to the social discrimination faced by people with disabilities. However, the field has not been so aware of the subtler discrimination that people with disabilities can experience due to the insensitive policies and priorities of the rehabilitation bureaucracy itself (e.g., Buchanan, 1996; Szymanski & Trueba, 1994). For example, the complaints of consumers have increased our awareness of the unwitting consequences of reducing to a diagnostic label the multiple dimensions that each person possesses. Similarly, the potential of clients can be squelched by our reliance on standardized tests that can pigeonhole individuals based on their performance on a series of perceptual-motor tasks or personality inventories. The impact of diagnostic labels can be particularly depersonalizing to clients in service systems that are based on a narrow medical model of identifying and treating pathology. Having an I-thou orientation that facilitates seeing the spiritual essence of our clients can help us counteract the stigmatizing effects of professional labels, priorities, and routines geared to the convenient operation of the service system.

Another commonality between counseling and spiritual practices is *self-examination as a process for maintaining awareness and openness to change.* Intuition is similarly respected in both practices. In contrast, most other areas of our culture so idolize logical positivism and the accumulation of information that other ways of knowing often get rejected outright, thereby reducing our access to wisdom. Our students gradually learn that effective counseling requires achieving a delicate balance between (a) application of micro-skills and (b) the art of being and responding in the here and now. We devote considerable curriculum attention to the former by training them to master the micro-techniques of counseling. Concerning the latter skill of being truly present, the students' intuitive clinical sense and reflective self-awareness are too often left to evolve, with the hope that these assets will eventually become integrated and accessible to them in the moment of need. Engaging in a personally selected spiritual practice like meditation or prayer to develop implicit trust in divine guidance, not just earned trust with another person, would enhance a counselor's grounding in the self and the moment.

There are also reasons based in a multicultural framework that argue for counselors to be open to spirituality as a dimension of clients and of the counseling process. It is fundamental to achieving multicultural competence for counselors to develop awareness of their own culturally shaped viewpoints and how those mesh with the corresponding viewpoints of clients. Because it is deeply infused within many cultures, religion is likely to be a contributing dimension of clients' background socialization and perspective on problems.

The best available framework for assessing a counselor's readiness to anticipate and respond to spiritual content and process is the list of competencies related to spirituality in counseling practice. This proposed set of nine skills was developed and endorsed under the auspices of the Association for Spiritual, Ethical, and Religious Values in Counseling (ASERVIC) and is reprinted in several sources (e.g., Morgan, 2000; Young, Cashwell, Wiggins-Frame & Belaire, 2002). See also Appendix A at the back of this book.

## Influential Experiences along My Spiritual Journey

The complexities of life occasionally bring me to pine for the ease of being comforted and controlled by the religion in which I was devoutly raised as a Boston Irish Catholic boy in the 1950s and 1960s. Otherwise, I neither credit nor blame my religious upbringing for the path of my spiritual search as an adult and a rehabilitation professional. Actually, I have been as much influenced by periodic spiritual experiences within my faith journey, such as dedicated retreats and workshops, as by the ongoing religious offerings (e.g., dogma, ritual) within my formal faith affiliations. In Erich Fromm's (1950) terms, it could be said that I have gradually moved from "authoritarian religion" to "humanistic religion." My own perception of the experience is consonant with how I interpret Artress's (1995) explanation of religion as the container and spirituality as the essences within it.

I have long been intrigued by personal metaphors for God or faith, such as confidante, friend, or light. Some acquaintances have described their appreciation of their religious faith as "like a rock" that provides them with a solid foundation for everyday living and with a refuge during the turbulent challenges of life. For me, spirituality is like the sky—amorphous and evolving, yet overarching and ever-present. I find it majestic, whether at sunrise on a brilliant, crisp day or during a sultry, stormy night. It is constant and yet ever-changing; bigger and more mysterious than anything I can concretely imagine, while also just being there like a backdrop behind the busy routines that march us through daily life.

A period of significant "spiritual formation" for me was the process of coming to realize and declare myself a conscientious objector (CO) at age twenty. I see its impact in three arenas of my spirituality. First, it was an enriching time of discovery for me. I was given both validation for being my pacifist self and an education about how to formalize that moral identity in my world. Being given these gifts by spiritual people who were either (a) folks of a different religion than I had ever known, primarily Quakers, or (b) folks of no religious leanings at all, helped to draw me out of the cocoon and tradition of my homogeneously Roman Catholic culture and background. Second, the process also had its episodes of the dark night of the soul. I had nightmares of being a CO whose application for official status as such had been denied by the Selective Service System and of then enduring a brutal prison term. I felt as if I were under scrutiny and suspicion, that my future was controlled by a bureaucracy that I saw as self-righteous and amoral. The third aspect was seeing spirituality in action through the work and lifestyle of the COs, Quakers, and peace activists I met during this time. This is perhaps the clearest connection for me between spirituality as an intimately personal resource and its implicit or intentional implementation in service to others, whether that be as a parent or a pastor, a caregiver or a counselor.

My awakening to spirituality and its potential was further expanded in a variety of ways. Most directly, I have been inspired by the words and insights of some famous authors whose spiritual writings I have read and whom I also had the good fortune to hear speak in person, albeit in large conference gatherings. These included: Viktor Frankl while I was a student in Vienna in 1970 (coincidentally, I heard this Holocaust survivor shortly after I had a powerful experience visiting a former Nazi concentration camp and meeting a man with a passionate personality who had been rescued from there as a child at the end of the war); Bernie Siegel at the American Counseling Association meeting in Boston in 1989; and Ram Dass at two workshops I attended. (See the References list for selected examples of their publications.) I have also been touched by more mundane manifestations of spirituality. For elaboration, let the following single example suffice. While living in midtown Manhattan and working at my first professional job, I found the adult-education yoga classes I took in a drab basement cafeteria of a public school more spiritually helpful and healing than the services at the variety of renowned and well-endowed churches I visited in the metropolis of New York City.

For approximately the past twenty-five years, I have been a practicing Unitarian-Universalist (UU; for more information on this denomination, see *www.uua.org*). To me, there are several affinities between this chosen religious path and my professional values. One clear connection is between the essential UU promotion of ongoing spiritual search and my own eclectic clinical orientation. Specifically, the fourth UU principle encourages "a free and responsible search for truth and meaning." UU services and literature reinforce this continuing search for the wisdom that has emerged from the world's religions. Moreover, UU encourages integrating into one's own evolving belief system those parts that resonate with who one is and how one wants to live in the world.

Similarly, my clinical approach strongly favors ongoing exploration of available counseling models and techniques, followed by internal reflection on how they fit the counselor's nature and the needs of clients. This approach promotes not only expansive thinking but also recognition that there is no single correct response to what clients express in counseling. Many students seem to believe that there is such a "right answer" to most client statements. Being spiritually open helps, I think, to develop a better sense of faith—in the self, the client, and in the process—that can liberate us from the myth of the perfectly matched therapeutic response. An added advantage of my UU-facilitated study and celebration of the contributions of the world's religions has been to increase my professional awareness and appreciation of client cultural diversity and alternative medical practices (e.g., McCarthy, 1997).

Another nexus between my spiritual and professional philosophies is represented by the active UU agenda to advance the causes of social justice and my own commitment within rehabilitation toward consumer advocacy and promotion of disability rights (e.g., McCarthy & Leierer, 2001; McCarthy, 2003). Many denominations make laudable efforts to alleviate suffering and injustice, but none in my experience matches the extent to which UU has disentangled its altruism from any motives of self-interest by not proselytizing the beneficiaries of its service programs. The sole purpose of the UU Service Committee is to develop empowering partnerships with small, indigenous, grass-roots organizations throughout the Third World.

## Introducing Ideas about Spirituality into Counselor and Rehabilitation Education

My career for the last twenty years has been primarily as a rehabilitation counselor educator. Therefore, most of the instructive experiences that I have to share emerged from educational efforts to advance consideration of spirituality, both as a component of rehabilitation consumers' lives and as an option within the service provider's repertoire.

On a general level, I briefly but regularly try to bring my attention (and often that of those I am with) to nurturing the spiritual side of the work at hand. For example, I aim to begin or end each class with a brief inspirational recitation. Typical readings communicate messages about gratitude, keeping things in perspective, or the amazing potential of the human body-mind-spirit. I intend this to be useful in the content of the words and the process of the ritual: to give students uplifting food for thought and to model taking time out to nurture ourselves as a community while still tackling the tasks on the academic agenda. With each new semester, I invite students to take the initiative at any time they wish and bring a favorite reading to share with the class.

Each year, in a survey course covering a smorgasbord of psychosocial issues and their connection to disability, I devote the three hours of one class to the theme of spirituality. The class includes three components. First, I give a lecture in which I elaborate the concepts that are summarized in Table 11.1. Then I introduce a few thought-provoking questions and scenarios, and students organize themselves into small groups to discuss their chosen one. I consider it especially important for closely personal topics like spirituality to be given discussion time in a relatively intimate forum for learning through peer exchange. The questions and scenarios are devised by the students; they are based on assigned readings on the topic and are submitted to me in advance so I can construct a challenging, varied selection. Each group gives to the class a brief report outlining the outcomes generated by its discussion.

For the last activity, I facilitate a group reflection. As I rearrange the chairs, I explain the ancient symbol of the circle or mandala and its meanings in sacred traditions. I demonstrate the use of a variety of tools and techniques (e.g., meditation music, candles, a rainstick, a Zen garden, a pictorial labyrinth) for creating a spiritually inviting atmosphere within the counseling room and process. The majority of students report that they have found this class very engaging and expanding, at least personally if not also professionally. A common reaction has been curiosity about, if not downright eagerness to learn, how spirituality could be incorporated into counseling sessions.

Many students claim the presentation was the first time in the curriculum (or for some, in their entire post-secondary education) that any aspect of spirituality had been broached. They explain that the permissive discussions during class served to lift some of the professional taboo they perceived about the topic. Still, they say it is difficult for them to imagine concrete ways to implement the concept within counseling. Furthermore, some fear that introducing a spiritual perspective would lead them inadvertently to impose their own beliefs or to be perceived as doing so by clients or supervisors. Even if not concerned about crossing into ethically precarious territory, others prefer not to complicate counseling by broaching a potentially delicate subject like spirituality. One benefit of the current book is providing students examples of implementation through the work of practicing professionals.

Another reaction that the presentation on spirituality elicited is also worth sharing. The fact that I clearly recall it after more than fourteen years is probably an index of its potential for providing a learning experience. While the implications of the episode can be discussed in terms of a few different issues, I share it here from the perspective of its impact on me as an educator, a "planter of seeds." No doubt my personal interest in the topic of spirituality gets communicated in my annual dedicated presentation. Nonetheless, I specifically attempt to make it nonsectarian, diversified, and simply suggestive. I do express my belief that there is divinity in every person; and I propose that keeping this fact in mind—especially with regard to clients who seem annoying or exasperating to us—would help us be more humble and effective counselors. In the journal that students are required to submit after each class in this course, one generally smart and quiet undergraduate wrote a note to me. It proclaimed that my lecture was blasphemous, in particular for saying that there is divinity in every person. The student minced no words and selected scriptural quotes stating that proponents of such blasphemy would meet with eternal damnation. During class, I did not perceive any distress on his part, nor did he speak about his viewpoint.

At times over the years, I have recalled with regret that I did not initiate a private discussion of his feelings or otherwise respond to his note. I do tell my students that I think it is generally wise to be cautious about approaching spirituality in providing individual or group counseling; however, with regard to professional discussions and consciousness-raising about the topic, I indicate that I am clearly an advocate. I continue my small efforts to get spirituality included on the map, so to speak, of rehabilitation counseling theory and practice. However, the experience described has given me more empathy for understanding students' ambivalent reluctance to open up their counseling approach to the potentially touchy topic of spirituality. It also serves to remind me that messages, especially on sensitive subjects, can be construed very differently from how they were intended. Instructors concerned about this might find helpful the several tips offered by Young (2003) for dealing with difficult classroom dynamics and discussions stimulated by controversial topics.

## Suggestions for Incorporating Spirituality into Rehabilitation Counseling Practice

At the outset, it should be understood that there is a wide range of available options for integrating spirituality into rehabilitation work— from proactive to reactive, from strategically selected interventions to simple ways of being present. Frame (2003) and Tan (1996) arranged their many suggestions into explicit versus implicit strategies. Fukuyama and Sevig (1999) discussed their recommendations within a conceptual framework of awareness, relationship, and interventions in the counseling process. I shall also use these three rubrics to organize the following presentation of ideas and options for implementing spirituality within rehabilitation counseling practice.

### Awareness of the Spiritual Dimension

At a minimum, counselors can be open to expanding their own and the client's holistic awareness of spirituality. This domain as well as cognitive, emotional, or physical factors can affect clients' perceptions of their presenting problems and possible solutions. This awareness grows just by being attuned to the unspoken manifestations of the spiritual dimension. It develops by taking advantage of opportunities to identify the relevance of this dimension.

For example, intake interviews implicitly acknowledge the potential relevance of other mediating factors by asking numerous questions about the client's background, current situation, and available resources. However, the spiritual side of a client's history and behavior is typically not included. There is good reason to check out its potential relevance in an appropriately diplomatic fashion, as a routine procedure and early in one's contact with a client. Marilyn Ganje-Fling and Patricia McCarthy (1996) suggested that counselors use the initial informed consent process as a way of preparing clients by noting the topics, such as spirituality, that will be addressed during counseling.

Whenever it appears that religious aspects may be affecting a client's issues in counseling, Worthington (1989, pp. 589–592) recommends a thorough assessment be considered. He suggests the following questions to guide that determination:

1. How formal should the assessment be?
2. To what degree is the content of the person's faith to be assessed versus the process of "faithing," or making meaning in one's life?
3. How is religion involved in the life of the client?
4. How mature is the client in his or her religious life as well as in his or her cognitive, moral, and socioemotional lives?
5. To what degree, if any, is the client's religion related to the diagnosis?
6. To what degree is the client's religion involved in the etiology of the problem?
7. Who is the client?
8. Is the counselor competent to deal with this client's personal issues and the religious implications for the client?

Several practical models for understanding and assessing "spiritual wellness" have been developed (e.g., Banks, 1980; Chandler, Holden & Kolander, 1992; see Westgate, 1996 for a comparison of these and others). Counselors could utilize such models as an informative conceptual overview or a source of specific strategies for cultivating supportive spirituality in clients.

Many persons with disabilities voice the consensus that in most cultures there is a pervasive, though rarely explicit, association of disability with sin and punishment. Even devoted family members and religious authorities frequently operate on unconscious assumptions that disability signifies that a person is somehow "out of God's grace." It is important for counselors and other advocates to be aware of and able to debunk or reframe the various expressions of this negative message. Mitchell (2002) provides a powerful account of his struggle with the consequences of this archetypal religious myth.

### The Counseling Relationship and Being in the Moment

Another avenue for opening up the spiritual potential of counseling is to deepen the authenticity of the counselor-client relationship by fostering additional ways of connecting and caring. There are several dimensions to this quality of relationship, but I believe that most of them can be captured by the phrase *being in the moment.* The notion of "being" recognizes that the self has several layers of expression, represented by the public selves of our projected personality in our various roles, and then at the innermost core the true self. A thoughtful discussion of this was provided by Fukuyama and Sevig:

> it is helpful when counselors can reach into their own true being . . . when counselors can free themselves "to be" and not fall back on the safer routes of "doing" and "saying." . . . One way this plays itself out is in the relationship between two people and developing a "presence" (Korb, 1988). . . .The challenge becomes how to translate this process into the counseling session or, indeed, into life itself. . . . As counselors learn to listen to themselves and to others more deeply, access to this level of "true self" becomes more fully realized. . . .There are specific techniques that help access this source—various forms of meditation, breathing techniques, and exercises in grounding and centering.    (1999, pp. 143–144)

Developing the awareness and skill of being in the moment requires us to re-conceptualize time and our appreciation of it. Ram Dass has been a popular guru on this topic for more than three decades. He created a career out of his persistent personal journey toward enlightenment, splitting his time (but not his focus) between an ascetic maharishi who meditated in the burial grounds of India and the devotees of the human potential movement in posh California communities, then synthesizing and packaging for Western audiences the messages he absorbed. His tenth and latest book, *Still Here: Embracing Aging, Changing, and Dying* (2000), is another compilation of his personal experiences in conscious living in the moment.

The relevant twist in this publication is that, having turned seventy, he is now a genuine elder and since 1997 a stroke survivor whom doctors had given only a 10 percent chance of living after his cerebral hemorrhage. He discusses the differences among chronological, psychological, and cultural time; and he cogently bemoans our society's engrained "time is money" attitude.

> The more deeply we practice the path of wisdom, and explore the Soul level of our beings, the more aware we become of how little attention our culture pays to sacredness as an aspect of everyday life. . . . We're given to understand that time is something "spent" or "wasted," something we "have" or "don't have," like other material possessions. How rarely do we think of time as sacred, or the moment as a spiritual gift.    (Ram Dass, 2000, p. 141)

Most people today have been socialized to work and play at a hectic pace. Learning to live in the moment and to radiate that focused serenity on the job, even in the relative seclusion of a counseling room, can be an enormous challenge to our way of "being."

## Spiritually Based Interventions

Fortunately, there are hundreds of publications and audiovisual materials available that counselors could use to develop their skills in performing and demonstrating spiritually based interventions like meditation and other centering techniques. Many of them provide exercises that could be readily incorporated into a counseling session and/or used to teach clients how to practice these skills on their own. Clark (1995, pp. 161–162) offered a succinct summary of Buddhist philosophy that underpins sitting meditation and the ways it has proven useful to him in coping with the consequences of physical disability. This is one of his explanations:

> Society's conventional wisdom is that the best thing a disabled person can do is to try to become as "normal" as possible. This approach contains within it the implicit assumption that the disabled person will never fully arrive. Meditation calls into question much of what passes as normalcy. . . . Acceptance of the actual situation ("things-as-they-are" in the traditional Buddhist phrase) brings with it a kind of equanimity that permits a clearer assessment of one's options. . . . Compassion is the highest good in Buddhism, turning the focus away from one's individual situation towards that of society at large. . . . But changing one's outlook involves more than a simple act of will or leap of faith—it takes work. Meditation is a powerful tool for doing that work.

Mindfulness meditation and other Buddhist principles were likewise used by Walker and Walker (1995) to examine the problem of "loss of relatedness" in the counselor's relationship with the client.

Promoting relationships with experienced peers represents an effective clinical tool for nurturing rehabilitation clients' positive identity as a person with a disability while pragmatically supporting their healing journeys. Counselors should be enterprising about developing networks of individuals and self-help organizations to whom they could refer more recently disabled individuals for purposes of practical learning and affirmative socialization about living with a disability. The constellation of community-based Independent Living Centers that have grown out of the disability rights movement over the past three decades offers a prime source for initiating such relationships. In addition to these opportunities for direct interchange, bibliotherapy remains a surrogate means for fostering spiritual development in clients through targeted reading. Like many youth, my soul was forever touched by reading the spiritually infused autobiographies of Anne Frank and Helen Keller. There are numerous books about other magnanimous (though less widely known) characters who used their experience of disability or dis-advantagement for personal transformation and societal enrichment.

One role model of spiritual manifestation is the story of the disability and human rights activist Justin Dart, Jr. The grandson of a prominent millionaire, Justin was destined for an elite life of privilege. At age eighteen, instead of enrollment at an expensive prep school, fate gave him a very different growth experience: contracting polio and being described by a doctor as "better off dead than crippled for life" ("Empowerment," 1998, p. 18). Eventually, he abandoned his lucrative position and lifestyle as a corporate CEO, so that he and his wife Yoshiko could experience an ascetic life of retreat for six years in a primitive cabin in the Japanese mountains. During that time, he purged himself of his addictions to alcohol and prescription drugs; he grew in consciousness and contemplated how to fight the addictions of society (to money, power, and prestige) that cause oppression and other social evils. For decades, he and Yoshiko conducted their own version of foster parenting that they called "life-quality training." They sponsored more than eighty international youth (many of whom had disabilities) and mentored them in their home, providing them with the supports and skills training to start working and living independently. A biographical account of Justin's spirited life and advocacy work is one of the chapters in *Enabling Lives: Biographies of Six Prominent Americans with Disabilities* (McMahon & Shaw, 2000). This is but one example of a book that could be recommended for bibliotherapy as an adjunct to rehabilitation counseling.

Embracing spiritual practice may be our best hope not only for achieving a meaningful counselor-client relationship, but also for promoting wellness of body, mind, and spirit. Power in the spiritual realm is derived from metaphysical sources through personal consciousness and practices such as verbal affirmation and visual imagery. The field of psychoneuroimmunology (e.g., Ader, Felten & Cohen, 1991; Borysenko, 1993; Chopra, 1989) has investigated and demonstrated, through traditional scientific methods, some influences of these metaphysical practices and energy on a variety of physical phenomena, such as tumor growth and immune system function, not just on mental states. Although these metaphysical processes may require practice and guidance to perfect, it is important to acknowledge that these methods are (a) often useful even in their uncultivated state, (b) always available, and (c) independently accessible to each person, regardless of physical limitations, socioeconomic status, or other potentially constraining characteristics.

## Caveats about Integrating Spirituality into Counseling

Foremost to mention is the general tenet that clients should not be led down a path of exploration where they do not wish to go. Sometimes there can be a fine line between supporting a client to take risks in her or his self-search and getting a client to take steps that she or he has quietly been unable to refuse. Bullis (1996) proposed some specific contraindications to introducing spiritual imagery in counseling. These situations are (a) persons with psychotic hallucinations; (b) persons who are having or have had a stressful spiritual shift, such as changing spiritual orientation under duress; and (c) persons who have experienced abuse from clergy or membership in a cult.

In their discussion of counseling persons who had experienced early sexual abuse, Ganje-Fling and McCarthy (1996) presented several cautions about broaching spiritual issues. Because I believe they have broad application as sound guidelines to follow in working with many kinds of clients, I expand on them here.

Given that the realm of religion is in general a sensitive topic for many individuals, *avoiding premature spiritual intervention* is important. Often, clients are troubled by immediate concerns that are better addressed at an educational or psychological level before deeper, contextual issues are explored. This also allows time for the likewise essential development of the client's trust in the counselor. *Respect for practice boundaries and the role of religious professionals* is certainly important. As with any skill or subject area, there is a range of counselor competence and comfort with respect to spirituality. Some counselors would choose to be conservative in judging their own capacity to be effective in dealing with spiritual material presented by a client. They would honestly admit this and would offer to help the client identify a more appropriate professional with whom to pursue those matters. However, even counselors experienced and confident with respect to managing spiritual elements need to maintain awareness of professional practice boundaries and make appropriate referrals. Worthington (1989) concluded that counselors tended to underutilize religious personnel in treating client spiritual and religious issues.

Another caution is to *guard against slipping into countertransference issues,* which is an ongoing background goal in therapeutic relationships. It is not unusual for people, including counselors, to have deep-rooted and judgmental but unexamined feelings and thoughts about spiritual matters. Fukuyama and Sevig (1999, p. 148) reminded us that "there is no substitute for awareness and examination of the counselor's own beliefs and values," and offered some specific starting points for this self-assessment: "What does the client say or do that triggers the counselor's reactions? What are the counselor's beliefs that interfere with working with this client? What current situations outside of therapy are affecting work with this client?" Obtaining training and supervision for effectively handling spiritual aspects, as with any content area within the counseling process, is the best preparation and arrangement for escaping potential pitfalls.

Aside from the above clinical concerns, there are paradigm challenges that must be grappled with, if spiritual approaches to counseling are to be widely adopted and sanctioned. Primary among these is a critical shift in thinking and values away from ego to the cosmos, away from intervention to transcendence. Fortunato (1982) offered interesting observations about the quite conflicting criteria of psychological versus spiritual growth that are worth consideration from the perspective of choosing a clinical direction. He characterized psychological therapy as focused on ego strengthening through increased self-consciousness, personal control, and autonomy. In contrast, spiritual growth is facilitated by ego surrendering through enlightenment, pure consciousness, and union with an ultimate source of life. Likewise, Gregory (1994) discussed the fundamental philosophical differences between traditional rehabilitation goals and those developed within the deep ecology movement and its influences—Eastern spiritual traditions, Native American beliefs, and minority viewpoints in Western religion and philosophy.

## Anger in a Spiritual Sandpit: A Sample Session

(The author is grateful to two colleagues, Dr. Stephen Leierer and the Rev. Krista Taves, for constructing this scenario.)

He had been a successful professor of classics at one of the most prestigious universities in the country. In each of the subcultures within which he traveled, he was loved and respected. Suddenly one day, he was hit by a car when crossing a busy intersection with some of his students. Six months after the accident, he returned to the rehabilitation hospital for an evaluation. After a morning of medical tests, his schedule ended with an appointment with me, the rehabilitation psychologist on staff. When he walked in, his face was contorted by anger. Indeed, his anger made my soul quiver because it seemed to command his entire being. I began with a trite phrase.

*Counselor:*    How's it going?

*Client:*    How do you think it is going? I'm blind!

*Counselor:*    You sound angry.

*Client:*    Damn right I'm angry.

[Silence]

*Counselor:*    Who are you angry at?

[Silence]

*Client:*    I'm angry at God!

I felt a little frightened because of the rage coming from the client. It seemed like the professor was attributing his blindness to God. Without the delight of his preinjury scholarly pursuits, he was demoralized and depressed. In this state he blamed God for his blindness. As I watched his nonverbal behaviors generated by his anger, I tried to tap into my own spiritual resources by taking several deep breaths, reminding myself of my spiritual resources, and allowing transcendent power to flow through me to help the client. As I moved between the client's pain and my spiritual resources, I received a quiet intuition: the man's pain is pouring out of a broken heart that feels betrayed by God. Counseling must access the professor's feelings about God and his perception of God's feelings about him.

Just as I had collected myself spiritually and emotionally, the professor blustered:

*Client:*    Did I scare you off? Where'd you go?

*Counselor:*    I'm listening. . . . It seems like it was hard for you to say that. That you're angry at God.

*Client:*    Well, yeah, I mean, how do you say that? God is supposed to be good, fair, just. He's supposed to do good things in the world.

Well, what could be good, fair, and just about what happened to
me? My career's gone. I have no future. I'm always going to be
blind. Everything I did is gone.

*Counselor:*   Sounds like you're blaming God for that.

*Client:*   I guess it does. I mean, is that alright? I can't believe I'm asking that question. I mean, I'm sitting here thinking about God,
and I don't like the guy. Is it alright to blame God?

*Counselor:*   You're wondering if it's all right to be angry at God?

*Client:*   Well, yeah. How do you show anger at God. God is supposed
to be love, forgiveness, all that stuff. But if this is the kind of crap
he let's happen, God's a . . . a Monster!

*Counselor:*   What's it like for you to think about God as a monster?

*Client:*   [long pause] Really frightening. I need to feel connected to
God, but I don't know if I want to connect.

*Counselor:*   Do you have a metaphor for that? Is God a punching bag
or tackling dummy? A rock? What's the image in your mind that
you are pounding your fist against?

*Client:*   God is a high jump pit. One who is able to absorb emotion,
attitude, or behavior without judgment.

*Counselor:*   So you see God as supportive of your anger.

*Client:*   Yeah. I guess so. It sure doesn't seem very transcendent. It
seems blasphemous for a mere mortal to be kicking and hollering
at God.

*Counselor:*   Who says you can't be angry at God? It seems like that
might be reasonable, given all you've been through. So what are some
of the things you are angry about? Let's talk about some of them.

*Client:*   I'm angry because I can't see, I can't read, I can't move around
on my own. I can't interact with my family as I used to. I'm not respected in my department anymore; people feel sorry for me. I feel
useless. Everything is difficult; everything is harder, simple tasks
take forever. I'm angry because God has made my life a lot harder
than it used to be. It's not fair. I want life to be fair. I want it to
make sense. Why can't life be fair? Why did God let this happen
to me? I was doing something good. I was a good person. How
could something so awful come out of what was supposed to be—
what should have been viewed as—a good deed?

*Counselor:*   Wow! That's a lot. It seems like living in the world is a
very difficult task for *you* now. How are you getting through?

*Client:*   I've got to make sense of this accident and my blindness. I'm screaming at God, trying to figure out these questions until I can't scream any more.

*Counselor:*   What are you screaming?

*Client:*   It's not fair; it's not just. God, you're just a puppeteer pulling the strings. You'd have more friends if you weren't mean to the ones you have. I'm not an object lesson for people. If you think you're going to use me to glorify yourself, you'd better think again.

*Counselor:*   Sounds like you're in God's face. Does God ever talk back?

*Client:*   Yeah. And then he makes me really mad because sometimes he's a smart aleck or a drill sergeant. And sometimes he's self-righteous, thinks he's better than I am. And I'm tired of life being one big lesson. I'm tired of listening to those people who got hit by a hurricane saying with calm acceptance that it's God's plan. It's my hurricane now, and I hate it. Why didn't I die? It's better to be a martyr than disabled like me.

*Counselor:*   To me, it seems like you've made the ultimate sacrifice. You've lost so much, and still life hasn't given you a break. Your road hasn't gotten easier. It seems like you have fewer resources to make a longer trip. That's got to feel heavy, overwhelming, maybe even impossible.

*Client:*   It seems like you're saying it's okay that it's overwhelming and impossible. It seems like you're saying it might be okay to say that God could be responsible. Or for me to want some sort of answer— and I haven't gotten answers, all I've gotten is silence. I'd rather God yell at me than be silent. I'd rather understand than be isolated, than not know.

*Counselor:*   It sounds like the darkness is pretty overpowering, too. Because not only is there a physical darkness, but I wonder if you're also feeling a spiritual darkness, when you are reaching out to God. What would you like to have happen when you're screaming at God?

*Client:*   I'd like God to hug me. Yeah . . . I'd like a hug from God. I don't want a "To Do List." I want a hug from God. It would mean a lot if I knew God cared about me.

*Counselor:*   Let's try this: Imagine that you're surrounded by peace. You're being cradled by God. You're in God's hands. I know that may be difficult for you to do, but try.

*Client:*   It feels awkward. I can only hold it for a few seconds before I start getting angry.

*Counselor:*   That's fine; that's a pretty normal response. Let's just try
it for a few seconds, until it feels uncomfortable and stop. Okay.
Then take a few deep breaths and try thinking about a nurturing
view of God holding you until it feels uncomfortable, then stop.

It is not uncommon for people experiencing illness and disability to
find that their old theologies no longer work. This client functioned with
a theology of reward and punishment. Being a good person meant that
God would be good to him; being bad would invite God's punishment.
Physical disability can then easily be transformed into an indicator of
punishment from God for wrongdoing.

Clients using this theology may quickly blame both themselves and
God for their physical condition. Because this client believed in God as
a punishing God, he feared that his anger would lead to more punishment. The therapist here is supporting the client in developing a more
open theology that helps him reconnect with his God. Had the therapist
been uncomfortable moving in this spiritual direction, the client would
have lost a valuable opportunity for healing and growth.

## Concluding Thoughts

Within the health care professions, I would judge that nursing has
made the most diverse theoretical advancements and practical contributions in promoting consideration of the role of spirituality. Therefore,
persons interested in its relationship to disability or chronic illness
would be wise to delve into the nursing literature (e.g., Barnum, 2003;
O'Brien, 2003). Another prominent source of publications grounded
in spirituality is the field of addictions treatment (e.g., Miller, 1997;
Morgan & Jordan, 1999).

Within rehabilitation counseling, there are many good first-person
accounts of dealing with a disability, all of which take an explicit spiritual focus but utilize varied strategies and theologies. Examples of such
publications include Elie (1995), Lane (1995), Levy (1995), and Nosek
(1995). Another set of useful sources explains and exemplifies how to
incorporate spiritual dimensions into a particular clinical approach.
Representatives of this type of publication are Curtis and Davis (1999;
multimodal therapy) and Hinterkopf (1998; experiential focusing
method); several techniques are discussed by Curtis and Glass (2002),
Richards and Bergen (1997), and Trieschmann (2001).

A third bibliographic category relates the professional perspective in
working from a spiritual stance with a person with a disability (e.g.,

Halstead, 2000; Priester, 2000; Ingersoll, 2000; Royce-Davis, 2000). Spaniol, Gagne, and Koehler (1999) presented a cogent analysis of the components of recovery from mental illness. Their conceptual framework of psychiatric rehabilitation—including the individual's reclaiming of power, meaning, and hope—encourages integration of spiritual perspectives into counseling strategies that would advance these goals. Many respected journals in counseling and health services publish an occasional conceptual or research article on the relationship between disability and spirituality (e.g., Riley et al., 1998; Roberts, Kiselica & Fredrickson, 2002; Tate & Forchheimer, 2002). Even more learning options are available through conferences, seminars, and workshops on spirituality that continue to increase in scope and depth.

I shall end by noting one final opportunity for using spiritual perspectives to make a positive impact in the area of physical and mental health. That is the dire need to create worldwide consciousness and community commitment for stopping the spiral of violence from crime and war that wreaks so much despair and devastation. There are numerous faith-based peace organizations (e.g., Fellowship of Reconciliation, Pax Christi) and counselor-oriented publications (e.g., Gerstein & Moeschberger, 2003) that can provide the necessary direction and inspiration to get involved in this sacred mission for peace with justice and dignity.

## References

Ader, R., Felten, D., & Cohen, N. (1991). *Psychoneuroimmunology* (2nd ed.). New York: Academic Press.

Artress, L. (1995). *Walking a sacred path.* New York: Riverhead Books.

Banks, R. (1980). Health and spiritual dimensions: Relationships and implications for professional preparation programs. *Journal of School Health, 50,* 195–202.

Barnum, B. (2003). *Spirituality in nursing: From traditional to New Age.* New York: Springer Publishing Co.

Baskin, T., & Enright, R. (2004). Intervention studies on forgiveness: A meta-analysis. *Journal of Counseling & Development, 82*(1), 79–90.

Beck, R. (1999). Encouragement as a vehicle to empowerment in counseling: An existential perspective. In R. Marinelli & A. Dell Orto (Eds.), *The psychological and social impact of disability* (4th ed., pp. 329–339). New York: Springer Publishing Co.

Borysenko, J. (1993). *Fire in the soul: A new psychology of spiritual optimism.* New York: Warner Books.

Bruno, R. (1999, November). Buddhism plus disability: One "step" closer to Nirvana. *New Mobility,* pp. 32–39.

Buchanan, S. (1996). Surviving a system: One woman's experience of disability and health care. *Rehabilitation Digest, 26*(3), 7–10.

Bullis, R. (1996). *Spirituality in social work practice.* Washington, DC: Taylor & Francis.

Chandler, C. K., Holden, J. M., & Kolander, C. A. (1992). Counseling for spiritual wellness: Theory and practice. *Journal of Counseling & Development, 71,* 168–175.

Chopra, D. (1989). *Quantum healing: Exploring the frontiers of mind/body medicine.* New York: Bantam Books.

Clark, W. (1995). Buddhism and the spiritually challenged. *Rehabilitation Education, 9*(2 & 3), 159–162.

Curtis, R., & Davis, K. (1999). Spirituality and multimodal therapy: A practical approach to incorporating spirituality in counseling. *Counseling and Values, 43*(3), 199–210.

Curtis, R., & Glass, J.S. (2002). Spirituality and counseling class: A teaching model. *Counseling and Values, 47*(1), 3–12.

Elie, M. (1995). Be still. *Rehabilitation Education, 9*(2 & 3), 183–185.

Empowerment: The testament of Justin Dart, Jr. (1998, March). *Mainstream: Magazine of the Able-Disabled,* 17–26.

Fortunato, J. (1982). *Embracing the exile: Healing journeys of gay Christians.* New York: Harper & Row.

Frame, M. W. (2003) *Integrating religion and spirituality into counseling: A comprehensive approach.* Belmont, CA: Wadsworth.

Frankl, V. (1969). *The will to meaning: Principles and application of logotherapy.* New York: World Publishing.

Frankl, V. (1959). *Man's search for meaning.* New York: Simon & Schuster.

Frankl, V. (1969). *The will to meaning: Principles and application of logotherapy.* New York: World Publishing.

Fromm, E. (1950). *Psychoanalysis and religion.* New Haven: Yale University Press.

Fukuyama, M., & Sevig, T. (1999). *Integrating spirituality into multicultural counseling.* Thousand Oaks, CA: Sage Publications.

Ganje-Fling, M., & McCarthy, P. (1996). Impact of childhood sexual abuse on spiritual development: Counseling implications. *Journal of Counseling & Development, 74,* 253–258.

Gerstein, L., & Moeschberger, S. (2003). Building cultures of peace: An urgent task for counseling professionals. *Journal of Counseling & Development, 81,* 115–119.

Gregory, R. (1994). Deep ecology: An opportunity for rehabilitation counselors. *Journal of Applied Rehabilitation Counseling, 25*(2), 45–47.

Hafferty, F. (Ed.). (1995, Summer). Spirituality [Special issue]. *Disability Studies Quarterly.*

Halstead, R. (2000). From tragedy to triumph: Counselor as companion on the hero's journey. *Counseling and Values, 44*(2), 100–106.

Hill, P. C., & Pargament, K. I. (2003). Advances in the conceptualization and measurement of religion and spirituality: Implications for physical and mental health research. *American Psychologist, 58,* 64–74.

Hinterkopf, E. (1998). *Integrating spirituality in counseling: A manual for using the experiential focusing method.* Alexandria, VA: American Counseling Association.

Ingersoll, E.R. (2000). Gentle like the dawn: A dying woman's healing. *Counseling and Values, 44*(2), 129–134.

Kanner, A., & Kasser, T. (Eds.). (2003). *Psychology and consumer culture: The struggle for a good life in a materialistic society.* Washington, DC: American Psychological Association.

Korb, M. (1988). The numinous ground: I-Thou in Gestalt work. *The Gestalt Journal, 11*(1), 97–106.

Lane, N. (1995). A theology of anger when living with disability. *Rehabilitation Education, 9*(2 & 3), 97–111.

Larson, D., Wood, G., & Larson, S. (1993). A paradigm shift in medicine toward spirituality. *ADVANCE: The Journal of Mind-Body Health, 9*(4), 39–49.

Levine, S. (1999). Children's cognition as the foundation of spirituality. *International Journal of Children's Spirituality, 4*(2), 121–140.

Levy, M. (1995). To stand on holy ground: A Jewish spiritual perspective on disability. *Rehabilitation Education, 9*(2 & 3), 163–170.

Maslow, A. (1968). *Toward a psychology of being* (2nd ed.). New York: Van Nostrand.

McCarthy, H. (1995). Understanding and reversing rehabilitation counseling's neglect of spirituality. *Rehabilitation Education, 9*(2 & 3), 187–199.

McCarthy, H., & Leierer, S. (2001). Consumer concepts of ideal characteristics and minimum qualifications for rehabilitation counselors. *Rehabilitation Counseling Bulletin, 45*(1), 12–23.

McMahon, B., & Shaw, L. (2000). *Enabling lives: Biographies of six prominent Americans with disabilities.* Boca Raton, FL: CRC Press.

Miller, W. R. (1997). Spiritual aspects of addictions treatment and research. *Mind/Body Medicine, 2*(1), 37–43.

Miller, W. R., & Thoresen, C. E. (2003). Spirituality, religion, and health: An emerging research field. *American Psychologist, 58,* 24–35.

Mitchell, M. (2002). My journey to reconcile religious beliefs with reality. *Rehabilitation Counseling Bulletin, 46*(1), 51–53.

Moore, T. (1992). *Care of the soul: A guide for cultivating depth and sacredness in everyday life.* New York: Harper Collins.

Morgan, O. (2000). Counseling and spirituality. In H. Hackney (Ed.), *Practice issues for the beginning counselor* (pp. 170–182). Needham Heights, MA: Allyn & Bacon.

Morgan, O. J., & Jordan, M. (1999). *Addiction and spirituality: A multidisciplinary approach.* St. Louis, MO: Chalice Press.

Nosek, M. (1995). The defining light of Vedanta: Personal reflections on spirituality and disability. *Rehabilitation Education, 9*(2 & 3), 171–82.

Nosek, M., & Hughes, R. (2001). Psychospiritual aspects of sense of self in women with physical disabilities. *Journal of Rehabilitation, 67*(1), 20–25.

Nowitz, L. (2005). The case manager's role in fostering spiritual wellbeing with frail elders. *Care Management, 11*(1), 11–18.

O'Brien, M. (2003). *Spirituality in nursing: Standing on holy ground* (2nd ed.). Sudbury, MA: Jones and Bartlett Publishers.

Pargament, K. (1997). *The psychology of religion and coping.* New York: The Guilford Press.

Powell, L. H., Shahabi, L., & Thoresen, C. E. (2003). Religion and spirituality: Linkages to physical health. *American Psychologist, 58,* 35–52.

Priester, P. (2000). Varieties of spiritual experience in support of recovery from cocaine dependence. *Counseling and Values, 44*(2), 107–112.

Putnam, R. (2000). *Bowling alone: The collapse and revival of American community.* New York: Simon & Schuster.

Ram Dass. (2000). *Still here: Embracing aging, changing, and dying.* New York: Riverhead Books.

Ram Dass, & Bush, M. (1992). *Compassion in action: Setting out on the path of service.* New York: Crown Publishers, Inc.

Richards, P., & Bergen, A. (1997). *A spiritual strategy for counseling and psychotherapy.* Washington, DC: American Psychological Association.

Riley, B., Perna, R., Tate, D., Forchheimer, M., Anderson, C., & Luera, G. (1998). Types of spiritual well-being among persons with chronic illness: Their relation to various forms of quality of life. *Archives of Physical Medicine and Rehabilitation, 79,* 258–264.

Roberts, S., Kiselica, M., & Fredrickson, S. (2002). Quality of life of persons with medical illnesses: Counseling's holistic contribution. *Journal of Counseling & Development, 80,* 422–432.

Royce-Davis, J. (2000). The influence of spirituality on community participation and belonging: Christina's story. *Counseling and Values, 44*(2), 135–142.

Sachs, A. (2005, January 24). 10 questions for Deepak Chopra. *Time,* p. 10.

Seeman, T. E., Dubin, L. F., & Seeman, M. (2003). Religiosity/spirituality and health: A critical review of the evidence for biological pathways. *American Psychologist, 58,* 53–63.

Siegel, B. (1989). *Peace, love & healing.* New York: Harper & Row.

Siegel, B. (1986). *Love, medicine & miracles.* New York: Harper & Row.

Spaniol, L., Gagne, C., & Koehler, M. (1999). Recovery from serious mental illness: What it is and how to support people in their recovery. In R. Marinelli & A. Dell Orto (Eds.), *The psychological and social impact of disability* (4th ed., pp. 409–422). New York: Springer Publishing Co.

Szymanski, E., & Trueba, H. (1994). Castification of people with disabilities: Potential disempowering aspects of classifications in disability services. *Journal of Rehabilitation, 60*(3), 12–20.

Tan, S. (1996). Religion in clinical practice: Implicit and explicit integration. In E. Shafranske (Ed.), *Religion and the clinical practice of psychology* (pp. 365–387). Washington, DC: American Psychological Association.

Tate, D., & Forchheimer, M. (2002). Quality of life, life satisfaction, and spirituality. *American Journal of Physical Medicine and Rehabilitation, 81*(6), 400–410.

Thoresen, C. (Ed.). (1999). Spirituality and health [Special issue]. *Journal of Health Psychology, 4*(3).

Trieschmann, R. (2001). Spirituality and energy medicine. *Journal of Rehabilitation, 67*(1), 26–32.

Vash, C. (2003). Service: Its psychosocial aspects and psychospiritual context. *Rehabilitation Counseling Bulletin, 46*(2), 115–119.

Vash, C. (Ed.). (2001). Spirituality and disability [Special issue]. *Journal of Rehabilitation, 67*(1).

Vash, C. (1995). Choice. *Rehabilitation Education, 9*(2 & 3), 229–237.

Vash, C. (1994). *Personality and adversity: Psychospiritual aspects of rehabilitation.* New York: Springer Publishing Co.

Vash, C. (1981). *The psychology of disability.* New York: Springer Publishing Co.

Vash, C., & Crewe, N. (2004). *Psychology of disability* (2nd ed.). New York: Springer Publishing Co.

Walker, M. L., & Walker, R. B. (1995). Mindfulness in rehabilitation practice, education, and research. *Rehabilitation Education, 9*(2 & 3), 201–204.

Westgate, C. E., (1996). Spiritual wellness and depression. *Journal of Counseling & Development, 75,* 26–35.

Worthington, E. (1989). Religious faith across the life span: Implications for counseling and research. *The Counseling Psychologist, 17,* 555–612.

Wright, B. (1983). *Physical disability: A psychosocial approach.* New York: Harper & Row.

Wright, B. (1988). Attitudes and the fundamental negative bias. In H. Yuker (Ed.), *Attitudes toward persons with disabilities* (pp. 3–21). New York: Springer Publishing Co.

Young, G. (2003). Dealing with difficult classroom dialogue. In P. Bronstein & K. Quina (Eds.), *Teaching gender and multicultural awareness: Resources for the psychology classroom* (pp. 347–360). Washington, DC: American Psychological Association.

Young, J. S., Cashwell, C., Wiggins-Frame, M., & Belaire, C. (2002). Spiritual and religious competencies: A national survey of CACREP-accredited programs. *Counseling and Values, 47*(1), 22–33.

Zinnbauer, B. J., & Pargament, K. I. (2000). Working with the sacred: Four approaches to religious and spiritual issues in counseling. *Journal of Counseling & Development, 78,* 162–171.

## Acknowledgments

I would like to express my sincere thanks to some dear friends who contributed to the development and improvement of this chapter: Lekoma Akate, Yvelyne McCarthy, Helen Tuohy, and Carolyn Vash.

# CHAPTER TWELVE

# Spirituality and Counseling: The Dance of Magic and Effort

## R. Elliott Ingersoll

I tell my students and clients that life is a combination of magic and effort. If you put forth the effort, the magic usually meets you half way.

I am not claiming that there are guarantees, that life can be controlled, or even that everyone gets a fair shake. Some people seem to put forth no effort and get more magic than David Copperfield. Others seem to give 110 percent, and the magic moves slowly. I am not claiming to have some secret, esoteric insight. I am stating, based on my experience, that there is magic and there is effort. I call the combination of the two "life" and the process of tuning into the magic "spirituality." Since counselors' main job is helping clients get more deeply in touch with life, it only makes sense that they integrate spirituality into their work.

The most important thing for counselors seeking to integrate counseling and spirituality is to be committed to their own spiritual practice. This includes being committed to the evolution of that practice and your understanding of spirituality. Your practices and your understanding of spirituality will change and evolve. A continued commitment to a spiritual practice will bring about enhanced awareness. Enhanced awareness is what counseling and spirituality have most in common and, as we enhance our awareness, we develop and evolve.

It is important to note that the person of the counselor is a primary variable in the counseling relationship. Given that, your spiritual practice is as important as your counseling work. The person of the counselor is a primary variable in the counseling relationship; this calls on counselors for a lifelong commitment to increasing their awareness. With dozens of lines of human development in which awareness could be increased, it is not realistic to say counselors must increase their awareness in every possible line of development. It is imperative, however, that counselors integrating spirituality into the counseling process commit to increasing their spiritual awareness through a spiritual practice.

The notion of your own spiritual practice and your understanding of spirituality evolving through this commitment to practice is important but not frequently stated. As we evolve, our spiritual worldview frequently changes. That is one of the blessings (and one of the curses) of a commitment to spiritual practice, to spiritual awareness. It is often hard to let go of things we have outgrown and previous ways of making meaning that have helped us survive. The evolution is part of what I am calling "the magic" and happens naturally when we practice and reflect on those practices.

Ideally spiritual practice will integrate body, mind, and spirit, but remember: no other person or institution can pick the practice for you. Sometimes I think our practices pick us more than we pick them, and they evolve as we deepen our commitment to them: magic and effort. Being committed to a practice does not mean rigidly clinging to the same techniques or expecting the same outcomes. Commitment means engaging the practice and allowing it to unfold even if that unfolding takes you out of your spiritual tradition. If you are centered in the tradition given you in childhood, you must accept responsibility to regularly renew your commitment to that path. If you feel called to a new path you must take responsibility to immerse yourself in that path. Making conscious, committed choices is how you tune into the magic that resonates with you. Some of my own practices (that I will share in this chapter) have evolved and changed over several decades as my understanding of body, mind, and spirit has evolved.

The same is true for our clients in the course of the counseling relationship. In the process of counseling we guide clients through reflection and then to action in the world where they generalize what they have learned in the counseling journey. It is this undulation of reflection and action, this "spiral dance," as Starhawk (1979) says, that characterizes spiritual growth as well as the integration of counseling and spirituality. In reflection and in action the magic happens.

## My Entry into the Profession

My own motivations for going into counseling are a good example of how this might work. Initially, I went into counseling because I liked the image of myself as someone who was helping others. This attitude was not without its share of self-righteousness, some of which is related to my early religious experience, in which self-sacrifice was presented as something to aspire to. Despite this, I had very little insight back then into the power this self-image exerted, and my initial forays into counseling were pretty much a self-serving endeavor. Through counseling and spiritual practice, I have increased my awareness of this and grown away from it, although I have not outgrown all of my own narcissism.

When I began seeing clients, I slowly learned that there was a depth of humanity in each client that required me to open myself fully. Only then could I experience and understand them; only then could they more fully develop a trust in our relationship. To open up fully to clients, I had to let go of my narrow sense of self and develop a broader identity that connected me to others. In addition, to really stay committed to the work, I had to grow beyond my own self-serving rewards to understanding what it meant to really care about another's growth. This process was supported by my own practice of yoga and meditation as well as some good supervisory relationships over the years.

From a spiritual perspective, perhaps it could be argued that my initial self-centered reasons for going into counseling were my personal *shekinah*—that little piece of the divine in me—using my own narcissism to help me grow. While the attitude of believing in helping others began as a very self-centered one, under the influence of my *shekinah,* it has evolved into a broader identity that, on a good day, focuses my awareness on my connectedness to other people. When one feels connected to others, there is a natural desire to help alleviate their suffering. From this perspective I think that the creator of the universe uses even our most self-centered aspects for spiritual development.

## Spirituality as Belief and Experience:
## The Case of Jan

As I have stated elsewhere (Ingersoll, 1994), spirituality ultimately transcends and includes all defining concepts; it cannot really be defined *per se.* That said, spirituality can be *described,* and counselors need to understand the breadth and depth of the description to integrate it ethically.

First and foremost, along with Vaughan (1995), I describe spirituality as an essential, integral component of human beings that can be expressed in many different ways. This is important because I am asserting that spirituality, while it may be nurtured by institutions like organized religion, does not need them to come to fruition in a human life. My experiences have confirmed that spirituality is part of being human, so it makes sense to integrate it into counseling which deals with the whole person.

Let me emphasize that experience is much more important to me than belief. Put another way, the experience of magic is much more powerful than a belief in magic. While belief may play a temporary role in helping a person change, experience is the litmus test for any belief system.

One client that I worked with (Jan) believed herself to be a "sinful person." Jan identified as a Methodist and had attended the Methodist church all her life. She had many interpersonal difficulties related to suffering from Social Phobia. She interpreted her problems as evidence that God was punishing her. It took almost a year for her to discuss suffering sexual abuse at the hands of her stepfather when she was twelve years old. When her mother found out, she divorced the stepfather, but no official charges were ever pressed, and Jan always felt that she was the guilty one for tempting her stepfather simply by being a female. Our counseling work spent a good deal of time examining her belief system and how this guilt had been subtly reinforced in the sermons at her church.

The primary incompatibility that arose for Jan was between her understanding of what a personal God was, and the fact that so many people (herself included) suffered. Suffering was far more pronounced in her experience than any evidence of, or belief about, a God who looked after personal details and intervened to stop bad things from happening. Jan developed her sense of the divine as she worked through the memories of the abuse. As she engaged in the grueling work of recovery, she began seeing some magic.

Her mother was initially shocked that Jan brought up the abuse after all these years, but gradually became supportive and shared feelings she had never shared with Jan. These included her own beliefs at that time (1960s) about what it meant to be a woman and a wife, and how damaging those beliefs had been. Over a period of six months Jan and her mother grew closer. Jan also had a dream in which she (an adult in the dream) confronted her abuser who responded by jumping off a cliff (in real life the man had died ten years earlier in a car accident related to his alcohol use). The dream had a profoundly empowering effect on her. She interpreted these experiences as God working with her through the process of recovery.

Jan also became interested in meditation as a way to deal with her anxiety in social situations. Although she had been on medication for her anxiety, she was able to discontinue this after only six months that included her counseling and meditation practice—more magic as far as she was concerned.

Jan continued counseling for almost two years with only a few lapses where her anxiety was concerned. She spent a great deal of time reconceptualizing God and dealing with the guilt of her decision to leave her church. She moved to a different church across town that was much more progressive and open to diverse perspectives. This move took courage, since some members of her family saw it as a "falling away" from the true path. Jan, however, had the courage to interpret this as the movement of spirit within her. Her experience led her to these changes while she recovered from a very traumatic life event.

In Jan's case, we see her experiences and the courage to deal with them related to her evolution away from a second-hand belief system toward an experience of a personal God who called her to a different way of worship and a different way of living. One of the biggest risks of counseling is that clients may change, and others in their lives may not like the changes. Such was the case for Jan.

## Spirituality and Development

As a human construct, spirituality exists in all people on a continuum from an untapped potential to a full and glorious manifestation. There are several important descriptions of spirituality summarized by Wilber (2003), each of which is important for integrating spirituality with counseling. These descriptions include spirituality as a *line* of development, a *level* of development, an *attitude,* and as *peak experiences.* I will address each of these in turn with some short case examples to illustrate key points.

Counseling and spirituality, as evolving processes, are developmental in nature. Counselors should appreciate this as much as anyone, because of the strong developmental base in our profession (Ivey, 1986). Human beings progress through several dozen lines of development throughout their lives (such as sexual, spiritual, kinesthetic, moral, interpersonal). While we progress through these different lines at different rates, we always have a "center of gravity" that generally reflects where we are developmentally.

For example, cognitively we may have glimpses of post-formal operational reasoning, yet our center of gravity may be in formal operational thinking. Similarly, we may have glimpses of Kohlberg's universal ethical principles but for the most part still hover morally at the level that focuses on social contract and individual rights. Another example has to do with the development of our value systems. The "center of gravity" of our values development is important and relates to both personal and spiritual growth (Beck & Cowen, 1996). Our values evolve when we experience life events (including crises) that overwhelm what our current value system offers. In counseling relationships, clients often shift to a new center of gravity as a result of the counseling work.

One client I worked with (Edna) identified as a Jehovah's Witness, and her value system included a clear demarcation between those in her faith and the rest of the world. While recovering from surgery, Edna received a great deal of love and comfort from nurses who were outside her faith, and she was convinced that the love of those nurses helped her heal. This experience moved Edna into a sense of the human community far broader than those who shared her religious tradition.

Societies also have developmental centers of gravity particularly where values are concerned (Habermas, 1985). Often these provide the first images and structures with which we make sense of the spiritual journey and other aspects of life. Integrating the developmental images and structures available in a society is easier than growing beyond them. While the center of gravity of a society will draw a person up to that level, if a person tries to transcend it to a new level, the center of gravity can also hold her back (Wilber, 2003). I have experienced this in my own life when I grew beyond the Christianity of my childhood and have seen the same pattern in clients I have worked with.

Because counseling and spiritual growth can shift our developmental centers of gravity to new levels and because growth and development are ongoing, there is no final destination where counseling or spirituality are concerned. I note this because in academia and in spiritual/religious circles there is a tendency to speak in absolute, final language. Many times we forget the evolving nature of knowledge. We get caught up in the politics of lobbying for our own constructs and sometimes forget the search for truth altogether. As Hegel (1969) noted, however, spirit is always in progressive motion and giving itself new form. We must keep open.

## Spirituality as a Line of Development

The first description of spirituality is as a line of development (Wilber, 1997). While disagreement exists on how many lines of human development exist, most counselors will agree that there are certainly several including cognitive, affective, sexual, spiritual, and so forth. When we posit a particular line of development, it is better to think of it in general terms and not become too attached to the way it is labeled. For example, there are many uses for temperature scales and both Fahrenheit and Celsius scales are acceptable as long as everyone understands which scale is being used. The same is true of lines of development.

We may say that spirituality is its own line of development, or we may refer to moral development, faith development, or religious development. Again, like temperature scales, as long as we are clear about which line of development we are referring to, all the latter may be useful. Wilber has also noted that some lines of development overlap with, parallel, or depend on other lines of development. Spiritual development, for example, seems to rely to some extent on cognitive development, and spiritual maturity requires an ability to tolerate ambiguity similar to the demands of formal operational thinking.

Whichever construct we use to refer to spiritual development, an important note on development is that it tends to progress away from narcissism toward care for others (Kegan, 1982). Wilber (2003) summarized both Gilligan's (1982) and Kohlberg's (1984) work in this manner, stating that people typically begin with a focus on self (egocentric), move beyond that to a level of care that includes others close to them (sociocentric), and ideally move to a level of care that is universal (worldcentric). This is important, in that a true spiritual practice will move a person along these lines in some manner from selfish, to local care, and ideally to universal care. As we develop, we become more able to expand our concern beyond just the self.

One client (Jeremy) approached me to work with him as a "spiritual friend" who might act in some sense as a spiritual director (see Edwards, 1980). Jeremy was a candidate to the Anglican priesthood. While our counseling relationship was brief (we met four times and then agreed to a referral), two things stood out for me about Jeremy. First, he really was devoted to his spiritual practice of contemplative prayer and appeared to have been a dedicated practitioner for eight years. Second, Jeremy clearly had difficulty with interpersonal issues that arose in his life. While gifted in and committed to contemplative approaches to the divine, Jeremy was interpersonally handicapped to the point where he had great difficulty relating to those who were less mystically inclined. This also seemed to have stalled his progress in contemplation.

It appeared to me that until Jeremy found a way to relate better to others, he was not going to progress in his contemplation. While I was not trained in the Christian type of spiritual direction Jeremy inquired about, I did have a colleague with such training who also was qualified to help Jeremy address his interpersonal growth. Our four sessions really focused on heightening his awareness of the need for well-rounded growth. After the fourth session with me, I did at least feel confident that Jeremy understood that excelling in one line of development did not hold guarantees for progress in other lines and that the other lines required some attention if any spiritual development was to proceed.

## Spirituality as a Level of Development

The second description of spirituality is as a level of development (Wilber, 1997). Once we accept that there are numerous lines of development, it follows that most people do not progress through them evenly (Wilber, 2003). This explains how someone who is cognitively highly developed (a researcher, for example) may be poorly developed morally (the same gifted researcher may steal others' ideas to further his own career). Thus there are different levels of development that we all go through in any given line. This raises a question: Is spirituality the upper level of any given line of development?

In general, human beings develop (Wilber, 1996) from pre-personal stages (pre-egoic), to personal stages (egoic), to transpersonal stages (beyond ego). Despite traditional psychology's position that there is no development higher than the ego levels, the hypothesized transpersonal level has been supported by researchers like Alexander and Langer (1990), Assagioli (1965), Grof (1985), Maslow (1971), and Scotton, Chinen, and Battista (1996).

Murphy (1992) has extensively studied extraordinary aspects of the upper levels of various lines of development including kinesthetic, sensorimotor, and cognitive. He has also examined our higher capacities for love, pleasure, and dealing with pain. Murphy (1992), White (2002), and others contend that we have not yet grasped the implications of evolution for spirituality and how spirit may manifest in the evolving human being. This line of research has also been continued by Sheldrake (2003), who has made an excellent case that the human mind includes what he calls an "extended mind" and that this extended mind may account for experiences like precognition. In precognition, a person experiences knowledge of a future event before it comes to pass. Sheldrake's idea of an extended mind is one unbound by chronological time and thus one that would have access to those events most of us experience as in the future. Such a mind has been described in the mystical literature related to advanced meditation and is included in the abilities of those referred to in many religions as prophets.

Using examples of the higher levels of some lines of development, let us see if they seem spiritual. Consider the upper levels of human physical development. Whether thinking of the *siddhis* from the Hindu tradition or the *charisms* of Roman Catholicism, Murphy (1992) notes that these may actually be "emergent features of human development, as capacities inherent to the richer life that is available to us" (p. 172). Consider the level of compassion of Mother Teresa or perhaps the cognitive capacities of Albert Einstein. In each of these examples, the upper levels of development seem to transcend the appearance of ego-based separateness and unite those experiencing them with the species at large, the greater rhythms of life, and perhaps even the divine. In a way, the upper levels of development are like a shortcut to the magic. I have known two clients who were recognized as gifted in childhood. One appeared gifted in mathematics and the other in music. It is interesting to me that they both described their experiences in the respective disciplines in almost mystical terms. They both felt themselves "in service" to a higher, greater good that became manifest as they expressed themselves through their work.

Wilber (2003) has made the case that the upper levels of *any line* of development may be spiritual but, he adds, a person can certainly have a spiritual experience at any level of development. The key here is that people who have a spiritual experience will translate or make sense of that experience using the tools they have at their disposal. If they are only capable of concrete operational thinking, for example, they will likely make sense of that spiritual experience in a concrete operational way. This seems applicable to some children's near-death experiences of the type described by Morse (1991) or some of the different interpretations of similar nonordinary experiences. For example, some people report encounters with nonphysical entities and these are described variously as angels, extraterrestrials, or figments of one's imagination (Monroe, 1982). Despite this perspective, it should be added that there are cases reported where spiritual experiences appear to open up access to the upper levels of development in other lines (Piechowski, 2001).

An example of the latter is an eighty-year-old client I worked with in a nursing home setting who was dying of renal failure. One night he described having what sounded like an out-of-body experience, which is common among people who are dying. He claims he saw his body on the bed and then "moved upward" to a place where a being of light greeted him. He asked the being of light why he was in a nursing home, and the being told him it was to help him learn patience. The experience was ego-syntonic in that it was ultimately comforting. The client (who had an eighth grade education) said he did not know who the being was but assumed "it must be St. Peter or something." He related that as a child that was who he was told met dying people. This explanation seemed sufficient for the client as to the identity of the being. Of far more importance was the message that he was somehow learning patience, and this triggered several sessions where he reflected on how that was in fact true and how this experience had been a radical departure from the rest of his life. Again, the key here is that the client's interpretation of certain aspects of his experience reflected his cognitive line of development whereas actually processing the experience seemed to coax him beyond his current levels of development, cognitively and otherwise.

We must also consider that if the spiritual realm constitutes part of reality, then depending on one's developmental tool kit, it is possible that a person might misinterpret a spiritual experience. Similarly, if spiritual growth ultimately requires transcending our ego, then spiritual experiences that emphasize the relativity of the ego could be frightening to the person who is not yet ready to transcend his or her ego-based sense of self. Echoing some Christian mystics, Huxley (1954) has noted: "by unregenerate souls, the divine Light at its full blaze can be apprehended only as a burning, purgatorial fire" (p. 56). Bache (1994; 1996) concluded that understanding this dynamic may also help us explain things like frightening near-death experiences.

### Spirituality as an Attitude

Spirituality may also be typified as an attitude that people may hold that evolves as they progress developmentally. Wilber (1999) stated that attitude is one of the most common ways in which people understand spirituality, despite the fact that it is difficult to operationalize. I have had many clients, for example, who tried to cultivate what they consider to be a "spiritual attitude" focusing on affirmations throughout the day. These affirmations were designed to reinforce one's awareness of things like love, compassion, and openness. Is any one of these the "right" attitude if we understand spirituality this way? As Wilber points out, we cannot really say that the requisite attitude is love because at the spiritual level, love must have already unfolded from egocentric to sociocentric to worldcentric, and the same type of love is not present at each stage of unfolding. Wilber notes the same problems apply to using something like "openness," for openness does not appear fully formed but rather unfolds in a developmental sequence. So while some people may define spirituality as an attitude, it is difficult to explicate.

The way some people describe this attitude makes more sense to me if it is framed developmentally. If there is a spiritual line of development, then we might say there is also a spiritual impulse similar to the Jewish notion of *shekinah* or the small piece of the divine in each person. If the desire to express and experience a spiritual attitude is viewed as the impulse to grow in the spiritual line of development, then it makes sense that this "attitude" will evolve as the individual develops.

## Spirituality as Peak Experiences

While it is true that spirituality may involve peak experiences, these experiences must at some level become integrated more permanently, or else their influence will wane with time. Just as clients must generalize what they learn in counseling to situations outside the counseling setting, people whose peak experiences spur their spiritual quests must find a way to integrate these experiences to continue development once the experience fades. While peak experiences themselves may not show stagelike development, one's understanding of peak experiences may. As with spiritual experiences, discussed under levels of development, peak experiences can be interpreted (or misinterpreted) in numerous ways.

One colleague of mine has for years been a practioner of Wicca. In Wicca, there are several degrees of initiation that correspond to one's progress in the Craft. This colleague has shared with me several peak experiences that have occurred over her twenty years of work in this path and her journey across two degrees of initiation. Her first peak experiences occurred in her youth where she reported regularly having a feeling of oneness with nature. She quickly learned whom she should share these feelings with, since some adults in her life reacted angrily when she talked about them. One particularly vivid peak experience came in the form of a dream/vision at age twelve where a Goddess figure appeared to her. In the dream, she saw the figure at the end of her bed and upon awaking the figure was still there smiling lovingly at her. My colleague reports she got out of bed to go to the figure, who slowly disappeared still smiling lovingly, leaving my colleague standing bewildered at the foot of her bed.

Five days after this experience, she had her first menstrual period. At the time, she interpreted the experience as a concrete visitation from the Goddess to announce the onset of her cycle. As she matured, she came to understand this through Jung's notion of "big dreams" wherein higher aspects of herself used the archetype of the Goddess to usher her into the next phase of self-awareness as a woman and toward the path that has been a lifelong devotion for her. At this point in her life, she interprets such peak experiences as glimpses into the next levels of development where her identity expands to a felt kinship with all living things. Her spiritual path of Wicca, with its focus on ecological concerns and "harming none" is at present a good vehicle for her growth.

## Personal Narrative of My Path

What I have concluded in my forty-some years on this planet is that reality is complex, and complexity is our friend. A Buddhist priest who worked with me years ago told me that we have to approach reality with great faith and great doubt: great faith that we can come to a clearer understanding of things and great doubt that we could ever comprehend ultimate truths. This has been confirmed in my experience and, while it makes it hard to feign certainty and evangelize any particular path, it has served me well in learning about the paths and experiences of others. The main goal of sharing part of my history is to illustrate how I stumbled into practices for body, mind, and spirit that helped me tune into the magic I've been referring to in this chapter.

My spiritual journey probably began as a small child (similar to my colleague described above) with the simple awareness that I loved the sensation of air on my skin. I recall my four- or five-year-old mind made sense of that sensation by feeling connected to something greater than myself that also was somehow in me. It was a magical sense. I was raised in the Anglican faith where my sense of the magical was given names and forms through which it could be nurtured. At the time, I did not realize that these names and forms were only a small sampling of the ones available. I had considered entering the priesthood, but my mentor in the church pointed out that while I would be good at the mystical, spiritual duties, I would likely be a disaster as the head of a social and very "political" organization (all organized religious groups have political elements). I think at some level he also knew that my interests extended far beyond where any particular religion could take me and that, sooner or later, I would want to try framing the magic with some of the other names and forms available.

About the time I was finishing my undergraduate degree in psychology, I suffered a severe injury to the occipital nerve on the left side of my head. This injury left me with chronic, severe headaches, dizziness, and a sense of disorientation. While being treated with cortisone injections and anti-inflammatory medications, the relief was minimal. In an effort to attain greater relief, I picked up a book on yoga (Hittleman, 1970). Not only did the yoga provide a great deal of relief from the headaches, some odd changes occurred in my body within the first month of practice. I experienced a series of physical purges. This was followed by a change in the way I ate and felt. I seemed to go from desiring regular meals to being more of a "grazer," and I recall feeling almost lighter than air for a few days after the last purge episode. More magic. This piqued my interest so I began studying yoga with a teacher and did some seminars with my teacher's guru at his yoga ashram. These were powerful experiences that forced me to realize that the body must be fully integrated into any spiritual practice.

This was my first affirmation that there are what Wilber (2003) called ascending and descending currents to spiritual growth. The ascending currents urge us to transcend the material world while the descending currents urge us to embrace the divine, manifest or incarnate in the material world. The key is to strike a healthy balance between these two currents, which requires full integration of the body while at the same time the ability to transcend the body. This is the path taken in what are termed the "nondual" approaches to spirituality emphasized in Vajrayana and Vedanta (Wilber, 2003).

What I realized was that for most of my life I had internalized a negative attitude toward the body and that even my physical exercise was more designed to "tame the demons" of the physical and "beat it into submission." These attitudes were in part responsible for the injury described above. Yoga was the first contact I had with a system that fully recognizes the importance of the body yet works with it in a way that also helps one aim beyond it. During this time, I kept feeling drawn to rituals that somehow honored the body and included nature, but this was too threatening to me at the time, so I kept deflecting those feelings.

Oddly enough, while studying at a yoga ashram I discovered a book by Alan Watts (1968) on Christianity that had a profound impact on me. It linked the myths and rituals I loved so much in the Anglican Church to other spiritual traditions and showed how they were really representations of archetypes universal to the spiritual path. This was my first realization that there were many ways to classify spiritual experiences and that the labels in the Anglican Church were just one set of many. This realization was to herald the beginning of a period where my mind became more active in my spiritual practice.

That book led me to a course of personal study that broadened my perspectives about different religions and religion in general. I spent time with people from different traditions and took part in their practices as well. I was able to view the *satsang* at the yoga ashram and the practices of other faiths as similar in many ways to the Anglican liturgy

I had participated in for years. I also had a gradual dawning awareness that the organized church was leaving some of the best stuff out of the services—the practices designed to put you directly in touch with the Divine. Having spent a great deal of time in a diversity of Christian traditions, I found that this shortcoming was fairly common.

As synchronicity would have it, at this time the church diocese I lived in offered a three-year program designed for people in the church who wanted to cultivate deeper spiritual experiences. I was part of this community of people who engaged in year-round study of mystical spirituality and retreat four times a year in order to explore different aspects of esoteric spirituality, including those outside of the Christian traditions. This community had a powerful impact on me and assisted me greatly in conceptualizing how spirituality and counseling intersected. One of the things I learned was that the key to counseling and spirituality was development and particularly being able/willing to grow beyond the familiar. I learned very early on that attachment to the familiar was a formidable barrier to spiritual growth.

As a result of this community I also spent time at an Anglican monastery, receiving spiritual direction and engaging in contemplation. I had a particularly powerful peak experience at the monastery that was surprisingly "a-Christian" in its content. I was in the stone chapel chanting psalms at the office of Compline. There was the slightest hint of sunlight fading away through the stained-glass window across the transept, and as it faded I felt illuminated with awareness to the point where everything seemed to glow. In this moment I felt a profound union existing among all things. I was part of that union. This union was emphasized in awareness, in consciousness, and I felt at that moment that the most profound spiritual practice was the cultivation of consciousness, of awareness. As a result of this experience I decided to do my doctoral dissertation on a topic that would integrate counseling and spirituality, since both counseling and spirituality are intended to expand and enhance one's awareness.

The goals of my dissertation included finding a vocabulary for the spiritual dimensions of being human that transcended but included the vocabulary of different religious practices. To do this, I worked with a panel of experts representing various versions of Christian, Wiccan, Jewish, Ba'Hai', Buddhist, Afrocentric, and transpersonal paths. The outcome was that I became more convinced than ever that there was something about spirituality that, although nurtured by various religions, did not flow *from* those religions but rather *through* them. While heretical in some religious circles, I found that this realization was fairly commonplace for people who felt they had had direct encounters with the Divine. This understanding of spirituality as a potential in all people was indispensable to integrating it with counseling, but at the same time drew a line between my approach and those people who believe their particular religion has a monopoly on spiritual truth.

Before, during, and after my doctoral work, I continued experiencing increasingly intense urges toward ritual that was based in nature and the body. After years of deflecting this calling, and after considerable meditation and consultation, I began studying Wicca and went through an initiation into the Craft. This was essential to honor and hone the awareness I had going back to childhood that I was somehow connected to nature and that through nature all beings were connected. The fit has been a good one, and my practice of the Craft has profoundly enhanced my sense of ritual, sexuality, and ecological concerns in a way that the Christian path was not designed to. It has also been profoundly helpful in harmonizing many tense relationships in my life. Wicca generally helped me temper my very masculine identity and tendency toward agency, with a feminine receptivity and call toward communion.

However politically incorrect it is to state, I have to add that my awareness of the magic I've been writing about received an irrefutable boost from the use of psychedelic agents earlier in my life. This use, for the most part, occurred in controlled settings where the aim was to explore the subtle states that the chemicals made temporarily available. During these states, I experienced the interwoven wonder and humor of reality as it is and of the intelligence behind reality. The humor piece is still very important, and it constantly reminds me to avoid those grim and cheerless reformers who claim that the only salvation lies in death through seriousness. While developmentally, psychedelic agents are not for everyone, I did experience profound insights while using them. These sessions were only the beginnings, though, because altered states must always be integrated into one's life and ultimately become altered traits (Smith, 2000; Wilber, 2003). Without the work of integration, altered states will be lost in time like tears in rain.

To integrate the awareness and insights shared here, my staple practices for twenty years have been yoga and meditation. When I identified as a Christian, I used Christian images in both my yoga and meditation. Currently, I sometimes weave yoga and meditation into my Wiccan rituals, but more often than not I practice them daily without infusing any particular tradition into them. I am possibly the world's worst meditator; my mind wanders easily and frequently. What I have learned from these practices is that spiritual growth is like any other type of development.

It is a combination of magic and effort. Some of it will happen "on its own" (the magic), but that will not be enough to carry a person to the farther reaches of human nature. For that, we must meet the magic halfway with the effort of a concerted practice. As I noted at the beginning of this chapter, any counselor wishing to integrate spirituality into his or her practice must commit to a spiritual practice and stick with it. As your awareness evolves, you may find that different forms of the practice suit you at different times, but the key is to stay with the practice.

This summary is certainly not inclusive of all the different paths that have influenced me. My excursions into martial arts, Orthodox Christianity, and my meetings with rabbis of different persuasions have also influenced my journey and the way I conceptualize spirituality. The ecstatic states brought about through sex, music, and physical exercises have also played pivotal roles in my journey. Ultimately, though, what I have learned is that spirituality encompasses every aspect of life and cannot be compartmentalized. It really does take body, mind, and spirit.

What I have learned on this journey so far is that by selecting a path and practicing, you continue to open yourself up to the magic. And it just might transform you. Since the person of the counselor is the primary vehicle through which the counseling process is engaged, transformation of self means transformation of practice. Magic and effort, reflection and action, commitment and transformation: If you don't believe me, try it for yourself. Try it for your clients. You might be surprised by the magic.

## Concluding Thoughts

- Take some time to assess how your spiritual practices relate to body, mind, and spirit. Journals can be a good way to do this.

- How have your spiritual practices and spiritual worldview changed over the years? If you think they haven't changed, how have you integrated them into a changing world?

- List the overt ways spirituality relates to your counseling practice. Is it something you include in any introduction to your services?

- Do you do any assessment for spiritual issues clients may be bringing to you?

- Consider a more extended spiritual autobiography that addresses how your spiritual path has changed from childhood, to adolescence, to adulthood. Include both peak experiences as well as realizations about when you have reached a new level in your development.

## References

Alexander, C. N., & Langer, E. J. (Eds.). (1990). *Higher stages of human development: Perspectives on adult growth.* Cambridge, MA: Oxford University Press.

Assagioli, R. (1965). *Psychosynthesis: A collection of basic writings.* New York: Viking.

Bache, C. M. (1996). Expanding Grof's conception of the perinatal: Deepening the inquiry into frightening near death experiences. *Journal of Near Death Studies, 15,* 115–139.

Bache, C. M. (1994). A perinatal interpretation of frightening near-death experiences: A dialogue with Kenneth Ring. *Journal of Near Death Studies, 13,* 25–45.

Beck, D. E., & Cowan, C. C. (1996). *Spiral dynamics: Mastering values, leadership, and change.* Malden, MA: Blackwell.

Edwards, T. (1980). *Spiritual friend: Reclaiming the gift of spiritual direction.* New York: Paulist Press.

Gilligan, C. (1982). *In a different voice: Psychological theory and women's development.* Cambridge: Harvard University Press.

Grof, S. (1985). *Beyond the brain: Birth, death, and transcendence in psychotherapy.* Albany: State University of New York Press.

Grof, S., & Grof, C. (Eds.). (1989). *Spiritual emergency: When personal transformation becomes a crisis.* Los Angeles: Jeremy Tarcher.

Habermas, J. (1985). *The theory of communicative action: Reason and rationalization of society.* Boston: Beacon.

Hegel, G. W. F. (1969). *The phenomenology of mind.* Translated by J.B. Baillie. New York: Harper Collins.

Hittleman, R. (1970). *Yoga: 28 day exercise plan.* New York: Bantam.

Huxley, A. (1954). *The doors of perception.* New York: Harper and Row.

Ingersoll, R. E. (2002). An integral approach for teaching and practicing diagnosis. *Journal of Transpersonal Psychology, 34,* 115–127.

Ingersoll, R. E. (1994). Spirituality, religion, and counseling: Dimensions and relationships. *Counseling and Values, 38,* 98–112.

Ingersoll, R. E., & Rak, C. F. (in press). *Psychopharmacology for helping professionals: An integral approach.* Contracted with Brooks/Cole Publishing for 2004.

Ivey, A. E. (1986). *Developmental therapy: Theory into practice.* San Francisco: Jossey-Bass.

Kegan, R. (1982). *The evolving self: Problem and process in human development.* Cambridge: Harvard University Press.

Kohlberg, L. (1984). *The psychology of moral development.* New York: Harper & Row.

Maslow, A. H. (1971). *The farther reaches of human nature.* New York: Penguin.

Monroe, R. A. (1982). *Far journeys.* New York: Doubleday.

Morse, M. (1991). *Closer to the light: Learning from the near-death experiences of children.* New York: Ivy Books.

Murphy, M. (1992). *The future of the body: Explorations into the further evolution of human nature.* New York: Tarcher.

Piechowski, M. M. (2001). Childhood spirituality. *Journal of Transpersonal Psychology, 33,* 1–15.

Scotton, B. W., Chinen, A. B., & Battista, J. R. (Eds.). (1996). *Textbook of transpersonal psychiatry and psychology.* New York: Basic Books.

Sheldrake, R. (2003). *The sense of being stared at and other aspects of the extended mind.* New York: Crown.

Smith, H. (2000). *Cleansing the doors of perception: The religious significance of entheogenic plants and chemicals.* Los Angeles, CA: Jeremy Tarcher.

Starhawk. (1979). *The spiral dance: A rebirth of the ancient religion of the great Goddess.* New York: Harper & Row.

Vaughan, F. (1995). *Shadows of the sacred: Seeing through spiritual illusions.* Wheaton, IL: Quest.

Watts, A. W. (1968). *Myth and ritual in Christianity.* New York: Beacon.

White, J. (2002). Enlightenment and the body of light. *What Is Enlightenment, 2,* 92–94.

Wilber, K. (2003). *Kosmic consciousness.* Audio interview with Tami Simon. Boulder, CO: Sounds True Productions.

Wilber (1999). *Integral psychology: Consciousness, spirit, psychology, therapy.* Boston: Shambhala.

Wilber, K. (1997). *The eye of spirit: An integral vision for a world gone slightly mad.* Boston: Shambhala.

Wilber, K. (1996). *Eye to eye: The quest for a new paradigm.* Boston: Shambhala.

Wilber, K. (1995). *Sex, ecology, spirituality: The spirit of evolution.* Boston: Shambhala.

Wilson, R. A. (1991). *Cosmic trigger volume II: Down to earth.* Tempe, AZ: New Falcon Publications.

❧

# Appendix A

ASERVIC Competencies for Integrating
Spirituality into Counseling

*http://www.aservic.org/*

**Competency 1**   The professional counselor can explain the difference between religion and spirituality, including similarities and differences.

**Competency 2**   The professional counselor can describe religious and spiritual beliefs and practices in a cultural context.

**Competency 3**   The professional counselor engages in self-exploration of religious and spiritual beliefs in order to increase sensitivity, understanding and acceptance of diverse belief systems.

**Competency 4**   The professional counselor can describer her/his religious and/or spiritual belief system and explain various models of religious or spiritual development across the lifespan.

**Competency 5**   The professional counselor can demonstrate sensitivity and acceptance of a variety of religious and/or spiritual expressions in client communication.

**Competency 6**   The professional counselor can identify limits of her/his understanding of a client's religious or spiritual expression, and demonstrate appropriate referral skills and generate possible referral sources.

Formulated and published by the Association for Spiritual, Ethical, and Religious Values in Counseling (ASERVIC), a division of the American Counseling Association. Re-printed with permission.

**Competency 7**   The professional counselor can assess the relevance of the religious and/or spiritual domains in the client's therapeutic issues.

**Competency 8**   The professional counselor is sensitive to and receptive of religious and/or spiritual themes in the counseling process as befits the expressed preference of each client.

**Competency 9**   The professional counselor uses a client's religious and/or spiritual beliefs in the pursuit of the client's therapeutic goals as befits the client's expressed preference.

# Name Index

# Subject Index